A Treatise
Home Remedies

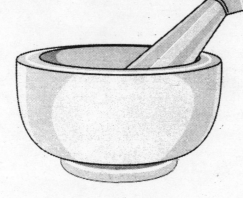

Dr. S. Suresh Babu

Edited by
Dr. Sunanda Sethi

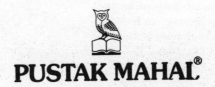

PUSTAK MAHAL®

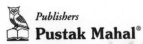

Publishers
Pustak Mahal®

J-3/16 , Daryaganj, New Delhi-110002
☎ 23276539, 23272783, 23272784 • *Fax:* 011-23260518
E-mail: info@pustakmahal.com • *Website:* www.pustakmahal.com

Sales Centre
■ 10-B, Netaji Subhash Marg, Daryaganj, New Delhi-110002
☎ 23268292, 23268293, 23279900 • *Fax:* 011-23280567
E-mail: rapidexdelhi@indiatimes.com
■ Hind Pustak Bhawan
6686, Khari Baoli, Delhi-110006
☎ 23944314, 23911979

Branches
Bengaluru: ☎ 080-22234025 • *Telefax:* 080-22240209
E-mail: pustak@airtelmail.in • pustak@sancharnet.in
Mumbai: ☎ 022-22010941, 022-22053387
E-mail: rapidex@bom5.vsnl.net.in
Patna: ☎ 0612-3294193 • *Telefax:* 0612-2302719
E-mail: rapidexptn@rediffmail.com
Hyderabad: *Telefax:* 040-24737290
E-mail: pustakmahalhyd@yahoo.co.in

© **Pustak Mahal, Delhi**

ISBN 978-81-223-0658-3

Edition: 2011

Printed at : Unique Colour Cartoon, Delhi

Dedicated to my beloved father
Late Dr. S. Nagabhushanam
(Ayurvedic Physician)
(1915-1985)

Preface

Even though there are numerous books available on home remedies, in my view, the term 'remedy' conveys a much wider spectrum of meaning than mere relief. It encompasses various types of measures to be adopted in the management of health at the home level.

The simple application or administration of homely available items or substances in a particular health problem constitutes only a fraction of this scheme. Unfortunately most of the books available overemphasise on this score leaving other equally important components like preventive, promotive, and drugless treatments, external therapies, positive health tips, diets, skin care etc.

Keeping all these missing links in view, this work **A Treatise on Home Remedies** has been crafted duly incorporating the effective herbal remedies for each common disease/ailment, which are widely used in *Ayurveda* since many centuries, without any side-effects. The combination of home and herbal remedies further helps in speedy recovery which are included in an attempt to make this work really a comprehensive and unique one among the series of books available on home remedies.

SPECIAL NOTE

Every care has been taken to include safe and harmless remedies, which will not produce adverse effects. However, as there are always exceptions to the rule, the remedies taken are at the readers' sole discretion, as even milk may cause intolerance in rare instances. When remedies prove ineffective, the doctor's advice is a must.

—Author

Acknowledgements _____

I would like to express my profound thanks to the many healers of India, who propagated the knowledge of home remedies and shared their experiences with others from generation to generation silently.

My special thanks are due to my student Dr. M. Madhavi (Post-Graduate Scholar) who has constantly encouraged me to complete the work and ably assisted in all aspects of the work.

I am also thankful to another student of mine Dr. P. Jyothi, PG Scholar for her help in gathering the information on certain kitchen remedies and preparation methods.

I also acknowledge the service rendered by my son, Mr. S. Naveen, MBA and wife Smt. Kalavathi, without whose cooperation it would not have been possible for me to take up this venture.

The chief inspiration for writing this book is the offer and opportunity provided by M/s Pustak Mahal, New Delhi. As such I am very much thankful to Sri Ram Avtar Guptaji, Managing Director, and Sri S.K. Roy, Editor of Pustak Maha! for their encouragement.

—Dr. S. Suresh Babu

Contents _____

Part-I
Diseases and their Remedies

1. ACIDITY

INTRODUCTION

Hyperacidity is a widespread common disorder which, if not treated in time, leads to ulcer formation in the digestive tract. It is mainly caused when hydrochloric acid, an important component of the digestive juices, is produced in excess.

TREATMENT

HOME REMEDIES

1. A decoction of sandal (*chandan*) may be consumed thrice a day for relief.

2. Tender fruit pulp of coconut may be taken from time to time. Tender coconut water soothes gastric irritation.

3. Simple sugar-added cold water also if consumed brings down the acidity level immediately. However, diabetics should refrain from this remedy.

4. About 200 to 500 ml of cold milk taken in sips during the day and at bedtime proves very beneficial in controlling acidity.

Causative Factors

- Excessive hot, spicy, fried food.
- Intake of fats, sweets, adulterated and fermented food.
- Alcohol consumption.
- Excessive intake of strong chocolate, tea, coffee, garlic, onions and excessive smoking.
- Stress-related conditions like anger, fear, worrying.
- Excessive exposure to sun and heat.
- Aspirin and anti-inflammatory drugs.

Signs & Symptoms

- Burning sensation in the chest and throat.
- Sour oral secretion/belching.
- Vomiting, headache.
- Heat in the body.
- Lack of appetite.

AYURVEDIC REMEDIES

1. *Avipattikara Churnam* is a good Ayurvedic remedy. 3 gm of powder well dissolved in 50ml of hot water, should be taken twice a day for 40 days.

2. Sooktyn tablets in doses of 1 tablet thrice a day with lukewarm water is another effective remedy.

3. *Sutshekar Ras* (simple) 1 tablet thrice daily taken with water after meals controls acidity effectively.

4. *Kamdudha Ras* (with pearls) is a drug of choice for acidity taken in the dose of 1 tablet thrice daily.

For details on Ayurvedic Standard Medicines, refer to Glossary

2. GAS/FLATULENCE

INTRODUCTION

"Passing gas" is certainly an embarassing situation as it is considered bad manners. An average person belches once or twice a day, especially after meals. In some societies, belching after a meal is taken by the host as a compliment. In infants, it is called burping.

On an average, an Indian passes flatus 2 to 4 times a day, and this gas is usually not foul smelling. Some people, when in company, avoid passing flatus, with the result that they suffer from abdominal discomfort. Ayurveda prohibits the suppression of this natural gas expulsion.

Technically, though, there is a slight difference between the gas coming out from both these orifices (i.e., mouth and rectum). In a belch after a meal, we expel air swallowed while eating. If a sour after-taste in the mouth follows a belch, it is a symptom of indigestion and it also means we are expelling gases formed in the stomach.

Only on the other hand, gas is always formed internally as a result of incomplete digestion. Food must be broken down into simple sugars and amino acids in order to be efficiently absorbed by the body. Complex sugars found in certain foods, however, resist this break-down process, perhaps because the enzyme that does this work is either weak or the person does not produce this enzyme. These complex sugars pass intact through the stomach and small intestine and enter the large intestine where they settle and begin to ferment. This fermentation produces carbon dioxide commonly known as GAS.

Causative Factors

One of the most common causes of passing excessive gas per rectum is incomplete evacuation of stools. Often this gas is foul smelling. Sometimes 'amoebiasis' may also cause the gas, and drugs like antibiotics also contribute to gas by changing the normal intestinal bacterial ?

Strong, high-fibre food, such as cabbage, whole wheat bread and beans which play beneficial role in preventing cancer, are often cited as CULPRITS in producing gas. It looks like the choice is between gas and cancer.

Gaseous distension can also be caused by lactose intolerance. People who lack the enzyme called lactase, which breaks down the complex milk sugar lactose, often find themselves passing large amounts of gas after drinking milk. Among others, greasy fried food, and pulses also cause gas.

DO'S & DON'TS

1. Avoid heavy smoking and *pan* eating/chewing.
2. Cut down drastically on your daily number of cold drinks and cups of tea.
3. Cut off intake of milk and sweets, if these increase gas.
4. Eat less than appetite demands.

5. Eat slowly, fully concentrating on the food, do not indulge in thinking while eating — this prevents swallowing of air.
6. Avoid onions, tomatoes, potatoes, peas, beans, dals and sweets in excess.

TREATMENT

HOME REMEDIES

1. Cardamom (*Elaichi*) is a highly useful home remedy. 5 gm of its powder can be taken with water. Take 5 gm each of fried asafoetida commonly known as *hing* (by frying in ghee, *hing* becomes pure), black salt (commonly known as *Kalanamak*) cardamom (*Elaichi*) and dry ginger known as *sonth*. Make fine powder, mix well and store in a clean bottle. ½ teaspoon of this powder can be given along with some lukewarm water 2 to 3 times a day which instantly gives relief from gas.
2. Similarly a mixture of 2 gm of *ajmoda* (celery seeds) and 1 gram *saunph* (anisi seeds) and sugar (as required) is given in doses of ½ to 1 teaspoon with lukewarm water. This also gives prompt relief from gas problems.
3. Take 1 part of *hing*, 2 parts of *vacha*, 3 parts of black salt, 4 parts of *sonth*, 5 parts of *jeera*, 6 parts of *harar*, 7 parts of *pohkar mul* and 8 parts of *kuth* and prepare a choorna. Take about 3 to 5 gm of this choorna twice or thrice daily with warm water for immediate relief from gas.

AYURVEDIC REMEDIES

1. *Hingvastaka Choorna* — can be taken in a dose of one teaspoonful twice a day with hot water.
2. *Hingutriguna Taila* — if given on empty stomach relieves constipation. The dose is 2 teaspoons once a day on empty stomach with a cup of hot water. This sets-in bowel movement.
3. *Kumari Asava* — an oral liquid, 20 ml with equal quantity of lukewarm water twice a day is also a good choice in gas problem.
4. Gasex tablets (Himalaya Drugs) in the dose of 1 to 2 tablets thrice daily with water is a good choice.
5. Ojus tablets (Charak) before or after meals taken 2 to 3 times a day give good results.
6. *Ark Pudina* (Liquid) or Ark Pudina pearls (Baidyanath) if taken give results within minutes.
7. *Gasantak Vati* (Baidyanath) in the dose of 1 tablet thrice daily taken with warm water is a good remedy for gas.
8. *Raj Vati, Lasunadi Vati* (Baidyanath) is also good for gas.
   All these measures, if taken properly relieve the problem of excessive passing of gas.

For details on Ayurvedic Standard Medicines, refer to Glossary

3. PEPTIC ULCER

INTRODUCTION

Any ulcer in the digestive system is known as peptic ulcer. This includes both gastric (occuring in stomach) and duodenal ulcers. These are very common in middle-aged men and women, who are 'acidity' patients for a long time. These ulcers are formed when a small area of the stomach or duodenal lining loses its natural resistance to the acids and other juices involved in digestion.

When this happens, the digestive juices and acids erode that weak point of lining and create a sore patch, which ultimately leads to ulcer formation.

Causative Factors

- Excessive hot, spicy fried food. Heavy drinking and smoking.
- Irregular, and bad eating habits.
- Regular intake of aspirin or non-steroidal anti inflammatory drugs.
- Excessive tea, coffee, and pan chewing.
- Gutkha is more dangerous.

Signs & Symptoms

- Burning pain or sensation in the upper abdomen or below the ribs.
- Some times the pain is felt after eating, but it can also be releived by eating.
- The pain may come and go over long periods of time.
- Some sufferers may feel nauseous.

DO'S & DON'TS

1. Avoid aspirin-based medicines, as they may induce stomach bleeding.
2. Stop alcohol, tea, coffee, smoking, *pan* and *gutkha* chewing.
3. Take regular, timely and balanced meals containing high-fibre food.
4. Above all one should be free from every day worries and tensions.
5. Pure ghee is a good ulcer healer, one should take it with meals daily.

TREATMENT

HOME REMEDIES

1. Cold milk is the best bet in complaints of heartburn.
2. Daily intake of 10 to 20gms of pure ghee with rice or meal is rewarding.
3. Banana fruit contains some ulcer healing properties. One to three bananas are to be taken along with a cup of milk. This provides a protective cover to the ulcer by neutralising the excessive acidity of gastric juices. However, the small yellow bananas are to be avoided and the larger greener ones preferred.

4. *Amlaki* - Botanically known as Emblica Officinalis, Indian gooseberry is highly useful and the fresh juice extracted from the fruit along with some sugar, if consumed daily on empty stomach, works wonderfully in this condition.
5. Certain plants which have astringent properties like *Patol Patar, Brahmi,* Aloe etc., are very useful in the treatment of peptic ulcer.
6. The decoction of barley, *pipal, parval* along with honey, can be taken for ulcers and acidity twice daily in the dose of 25 to 50ml.
7. The powder of *Harar* (2.5gm to 5gm) mixed with honey and *gur* has proved very effective for controlling peptic ulcer.

 ## AYURVEDIC REMEDIES

1. Ayurveda offers a wide range of drugs for this condition. One of the safest drugs that can be used regularly is *Avipattikara Churna* available in powder form. It is digestive, anti-flatulent and antacid. Regular use promotes ulcer healing by arresting excessive secretions of irritating acid and juices in the digestive system and throws out the unwanted toxins from the GI Tract through *Virechana* i.e., purgation.
2. There are other herbo-mineral and gold compounds like *Swarna Sutha Sekhara Rasa* etc., which are specifically indicated for this disorder. But they should be tried under the care of an Ayurvedic physician.
3. Vomitab tablet (charak), 1 tablet thrice daily before meals for 3 months cures ulcers completely.
4. Alsarex tablet (charak) in the dose of 1 to 2 tablets thrice daily is very good in curing acidity and peptic ulcer.
5. *Kamdudha Ras* (with pearls) taken 125mg thrice daily is another useful remedy.
6. Besides these, *Leelavilas Ras, Chanderkala Ras, Amalpithantak Loh* are other useful medicines.

For details on Ayurvedic Standard Medicines, refer to Glossary

Note : The doctor may advise tests like Barium meal X-rays or endoscopy to confirm the diagnosis. Initial treatment includes antacids and ulcer healing drugs. Surgery is considered if the ulcer leads to blood vomiting, or turns cancerous.

4. INDIGESTION

INTRODUCTION

Indigestion is also known as 'dyspepsia' which is a Greek term indicating indigestion or difficulty in digestion. It is a vague term very often quoted to describe any discomfort in the upper abdomen brought on by overeating. Most people suffer from it in day to day life, and it is often no more than a sign of overindulgence. Very rarely it represents a serious problem.

TREATMENT

HOME REMEDIES

The occasional mild indigestion does not require treatment and will be automatically relieved in a couple of hours.

Lemon is the fruit of choice in indigestion. The juice of half a lemon should be added to a glass of water, along with a bit of soda bicarb and stirred well. This should be taken in case of indigestion for instant relief.

Ginger is a well known home remedy in this condition. It stimulates the secretion of digestive juices so as to break down the heavy food.

Causative Factors

The term 'indigestion' itself conveys that food is being digested with difficulty. The reasons for this are many. Common ones include:

Over-eating, eating repeatedly, eating too much of rich, fatty or spicy food, which can irritate the stomach lining.

Other causative factors are pregnancy and stress. Occasionally, indigestion is a symptom of some other problems like peptic ulcer, gall stones or hiatus hernia.

Signs & Symptoms

The symptoms occur immediately after eating the food and may last for a couple of hours. Depending on the severity, one can notice symptoms and signs.

Vague discomfort and stomach-ache are common. Sometimes one may feel 'bloated' and 'nauseous'. Burping is another sign. Foul taste is an indicator of chronic indigestion.

Before eating a heavy meal, one should eat 2 or 3 small pieces of ginger, coated with a little bit of salt. This combination prevents indigestion even if one eats a bit more than usual.

Hing (Asafoetida) is one more dependable home remedy in indigestion. A pinch of *hing* powder and ghee should be added to some boiled rice and mixed well. This should be eaten before the regular meal, the daily usage of which ensures proper digestion and evacuation of bowels.

AYURVEDIC REMEDIES

1. *Shiva Kshara Pachana Churnam.*
2. *'Lavana Bhaskara Churnam'*—3 gm of these powders well mixed in lukewarm water should be taken twice a day.

3. *Hingvashataka Churnam* in the same dosage with ghee may be used before a meal.
4. *Arogya mishran* 1 pill thrice a day.
5. Gasex (Himalaya Drugs Co.) 1 tab. thrice daily.
6. Ojus (Charak) 1 tab before meals and 1 tab after meals thrice daily.
7. *Pancharishta* 15ml dissolved in same amount of water twice daily after meals.

For details on Ayurvedic Standard Medicines, refer to Glossary

DO'S & DON'TS

DIETICS

1. One should avoid all the factors stated as causative factors.
2. Certain eating rules should be followed.
   Do not eat and drink simultaneously.
   Do not eat in a hurry.
   Never eat to your stomach's full.
   Do not eat, when there is no appetite or as a recipe for boredom.
   Above all, the golden rule is that you should put your heart and soul in the food while eating.

5. HICCUPS

INTRODUCTION

Repeated, noisy intakes of air known as hiccups, are caused by involuntary contractions of the diaphragm.

Hiccuping attacks generally do not last more than a few minutes and are usually only a minor irritation to the sufferer.

APPROACH

Break up the sequence of these involuntary contractions and seek medical aid, if attack is prolonged or severe.

TREATMENT

HOME REMEDIES

1. Ask the affected person to sit quietly and hold his/her breath or give him/her something to drink.

2. If this is unsuccessful, place a paper bag (not a plastic bag) over the patient's mouth and nose, and ask the person to breathe in and out.
3. If hiccups persist for more than a few hours, seek medical aid or psychotherapy.
4. *Kulatha* in the form of a soup or dal is very useful for hiccups.

AYURVEDIC REMEDIES

1. The ash of a peacock feather is the best remedy in this condition. It is available at Ayurvedic stores by name *Mayura Chandrika Bhasma*. It should be taken in a dose of 5 gm six times a day, mixed with pure honey.
2. Cardamom is also useful, and the powder of one cardamom seed should be sucked with honey as required.
3. *Eladivati* is the drug of choice in this condition in the dose of 1 to 2 tablets crushed and given with honey 4 to 6 times daily.
4. *Sukumar Ghritham* can be given in the dose of 1 teaspoonful thrice daily with milk.

6. CONSTIPATION

INTRODUCTION

Constipation is the commonest complaint in elderly people, affecting seven out of every ten persons.

TREATMENT

HOME REMEDIES

DIET AND HABITS

1. Take plenty of green vegetables and fibrous food regularly along with fruits/juices.
2. Eat more *rotis* (wheat or *jawar*) and less rice.
3. Use whole meal flour, avoid refined ones.
4. Avoid fried items like *samosa, mirchi, masala* etc.
5. Above all, drink a glass of water in the morning.
6. Do some abdominal exercises.

Causative Factors

This is mainly because of lack of good eating habits like:
- Absence of green vegetables in adequate quantity and fruits in the regular meals. This residue material is essential to form the 'base' of the stool.
- Sufficient quantity of water must be drunk to keep the stool soft as the bulk of the stool is due to its water quantity.
- Reasonable time should be given for passing stool. Most people, because of a fast life schedule, give very less time for proper defecation. People staying in crowded flats, where there is only one toilet for 5-10 persons, also are prone to this problem.

Contd ...

7. Try to establish regular bowel habits and always answer nature's calls promptly.
8. Avoid excessive intake of tea & coffee.
9. Reduce smoking/drinking.
10. Avoid anxiety and worry.

AYURVEDIC REMEDIES

1. Regular use of *Triphala choorna* is a popular home remedy, easily available in Ayurvedic stores. 1 tsf with lukewarm water at bedtime is recommended.
2. Dry ginger powder & *senna* leaves' powder well mixed in equal quantity, is another popular home remedy. 5 gm of this powder should be taken along with a cup of lukewarm water before going to bed. This helps in easy passage of stools. *Senna* dry leaves are easily available as *sonamukhi* leaves at herbal stores.
3. *Sukhvirechan Vati* taken ½ to 1 tablet with warm water or milk at bed time, is recommended for constipation.
4. Herbolax tablet (Himalaya Drugs), 1 to 2 tablets twice daily for a period of 10 to 15 days, gives relief even in chronic con-stipation.

For details on Ayurvedic Standard Medicines, refer to Glossary

- Also if one makes a habit of holding on and not attending nature's call in time, in due course, even a full rectum stops sending calls. This leads to development of chronic constipation.
- Gastro Colic Reflex: This is the reflex phenomenon whereby, anything reaching the stomach, stimulates the colon, which results in a call to evacuate. Many people take a glass of water, a cup of tea, or a cigarette to take advantage of this reflex. Though this is not wrong, good eating and defecating habits are the only sure remedies.
- In women the tone of the abdominal and pelvic muscles is lost due to repeated child bearing. Most of the women do not tone abdominal muscles through exercise.
- Other common causes for chronic constipation are drugs taken for abdominal pain, hyperacidity, high blood pressure and headache. Strong purgatives also cause constipation.

Now-a-days because of aggressive advertisements in television many people indulging in daily consumption of some or the other of these purgatives do so, by making the bowel completely empty, whereby there is not enough material (residue) for a stool to be formed the next day. The patient, so, gets dependent on the laxative/purgative for the next passage of stool, thereby setting off a vicious circle.

7. CIRRHOSIS OF LIVER

INTRODUCTION

Cirrhosis of the liver occurs when normal liver cells are replaced by fibrous scar tissues preventing the liver from functioning effectively. This damage is irreparable and the tissue irrecoverable.

TREATMENT

HOME REMEDIES

2 tsp fresh lemon juice.
1 tsp crushed onion juice.

This mixture should be taken on empty stomach in the morning for 3 months to resolve cirrhosis.

AYURVEDIC REMEDIES

Ayurveda has been treating this disorder with a high success rate.

1. *Yakrut Pippali* is the drug of choice along with a herbo-mineral compound called *Arogya vardhini*. This should be taken under direct supervision of a competent Ayurvedic physician.
2. *Punarnava Mandoor* 1 tablet thrice daily with water after meals for 2 to 3 months gives excellent results.
3. Cytozen tablet (Charak) 1 tablet twice daily for 6 to 12 weeks.

For details on Ayurvedic Standard Medicines, refer to Glossary

Causative Factors

- Alcohol abuse appears to be the prime cause in a majority of cases.
- Chemical abuse, for example, over – doses of paracetamol, as well as cleaning fluids or anaesthetics, may cause cirrhosis.
- Hepatitis 'B' or glandular fever is a predisposing factor.

Signs & Symptoms

Early stage—Nearly none.
Advanced stage:
- Loss of sexual desire.
- Tingling sensation in hands and feet.
- Weight loss.
- Enlargement of breasts in women and shrinkage of testicles in men.
- Swelling of abdomen with characteristic fine red vein lines on skin.

8. JAUNDICE

INTRODUCTION

Jaundice is common in new born babies. It is the key sign of many disorders of the liver and gall bladder. It can develop suddenly or gradually.

TREATMENT

HOME REMEDIES

1. Sugarcane juice: This is one home remedy effective in the treatment of jaundice. Plenty of this juice can be given to the patient, to promote more urination as well as for nutrition and general health.
2. Barley water: This can be given, if the patient is diabetic, since sugarcane juice is contra-indicated in such people. This also causes more urination.
3. *Triphala* powder: A mixture of *Amla, Harada* and *Behada* can be given duly making a decoction. 20gms of powder, added to a glass of water, is reduced to ¼ quantity. This should be filtered and given twice a day.
4. 20ml of expressed juice of fresh neem leaves and 20ml of pure honey should be well mixed, and to this mixture is added 3gms of black pepper powder and stirred well. This should be taken in two equal doses, in the morning and evening. It makes a good home remedy for jaundice.

AYURVEDIC REMEDIES

1. 'Jaundex' syrup in the dose of 10ml thrice a day along with one tablet of "Nirocil", in many instances, clears the jaundice within one week. This should be used under a doctor's surveillance preferably.
2. *Punarnava Mandoor*, 1 tab thice daily for 2 to 3 weeks.
3. *Navrayas Loh* can also be given in the dose of 125mg thrice daily.
4. Liv 52 tablet (Himalaya Drugs) is a very popular drug, given in the dose of 1 to 2 tablets thrice daily.
5. Livpar tablet (Gufic) is also very good in controlling jaundice in the above doses.

For details on Ayurvedic Standard Medicines, refer to Glossary

Causative Factors

Jaundice may occur when the flow of bile from the liver, through the biliary system to the intestine, is blocked. The bile stagnates in the liver, which in turn means that the yellow pigment bilirubin, flows back in to circulation.

- Obstrtuctive Jaundice : Is caused by gallstones. It usually happens when the bile ducts are blocked and bile can not pass into the intestines.
- Haemolytic Jundice: Occurs when too much bilirubin is produced by the breakdown of red blood cells.
- Liver damage, as a result of hepatitis or chronic malaria may also contribute to jaundice. Alcoholism and poisons are rare causes. Jaundice is very common in healthy newborn bables, because of an immature liver.

Signs & Symptoms

The very first sign of jaundice are yellowing of the skin and the whites of the eyes, darkened urine and some times pale stools. The skin may become itchy before occurrence. The symptoms are exterme weakness, sudden loss of appetite, nausea and dull pain in the liver region.

DIETICS

Simple light liquid diet, like fresh fruit juices and a fat-free and oil-free diet is advised. Avoid *chutney,* pickles and non-vegetarian diet. Drink plenty of fresh and boiled water.

9. HEPATITIS

INTRODUCTION

Inflammation of the liver is known as 'hepatitis' in medical language. There are two important types of hepatitis. These are commonly called hepatitis 'A' and hepatitis 'B'. Each is caused by different viruses.

HEPATITIS 'A'

This is milder than 'B' type of hepatitis. It is more infectious and occurs more commonly.

TREATMENT

1. Drink plenty of water and other fluids like sugarcane juice, coconut water, barley water etc.
2. Take rest as it requires a few weeks to recover completely.
3. One may feel tired and depressed for some time; so rest is essential.
4. A high degree of hygiene is important to prevent further spread of infection.
5. Boiled and filtered water should be consumed.

Causative Factors

Hepatitis 'A' is usually transmitted through unhygienic or contaminated food or water.

Signs & Symptoms

The initial signs are fever and headache, followed by nauseating sensation, vomiting and discomfort over the region of liver, which lies under the ribs in the upper right-hand side of the abdomen.

After three or four days of the above stated signs and symptoms, jaundice will appear and gradually worsen over a week.

The affected person's urine may be dark-brown in colour. Generalised itching over the body may also occur in some. Recovery takes place in the next one or two weeks time.

HOME REMEDIES

1. Take pure turmeric powder, add 10gms of this powder to 50gms of pure yoghurt and mix well, and divide into equal parts. Drink 1 part in the morning and another in the evening for 15 days. This simple home remedy works well in many instances.
2. Sugarcane should be sucked three or four times a day. It nourishes the body and works as a diuretic thereby clearing the urine.

AYURVEDIC REMEDIES are same as in the case of jaundice.

10. PILES

INTRODUCTION

Piles, also known as 'haemorrhoids', are small, bluish swellings, comprising of enlarged blood vessels situated either just inside or just outside the anus commonly called internal piles and external piles. In case of bleeding, they are termed as bleeding piles.

Type	Main feature
Ext. Piles	— Severe pain/no bleeding.
Internal Piles	— Discharge of dark blood.
Bleeding Piles	— Excessive bleeding on bursting of vessels.
CONSTIPATION IS THE KEY FEATURE OF ALL TYPES OF PILES.	

TREATMENT

HOME REMEDIES

1. The poultice made of sesame (*til*) seeds can be applied over bleeding piles as an external measure, and internally also ½ teaspoonful of sesame seeds can be taken orally with some butter.

2. A mixture can be made of:
   Ripe *bael* fruit pulp   = 1oz
   Sugar   = 180gms
   Powder of black peppers = 7 in number
   Cardamom powder   = 7gms
   This can be taken twice a day as a good remedy.

3. Radish (*Muli*) is a useful home remedy for piles.
   * The hot poultice of dry radish (*Muli*) is a good application in non-bleeding piles.
   * The juice is also useful in piles. 60 to 100 ml of radish juice well mixed with little bit of salt, should be taken twice a day, daily for 40 days.

Causative Factors

- Persistent constipation due to poor dietary habits.
- Sitting on hard seats for prolonged periods.
- Lack of exercise.

Because of all these factors, straining is needed to pass the small hard stools, which causes congestion in the network of blood vessels located inside the anal cushions. Gradually, these vessels enlarge and form piles. If the constipation further continues, they become large enough to be called second or third degree piles.

Signs & Symptoms

Internal or First-degree Piles: Many people have these without even being aware of them. These are located just inside the anus, ocassionally causing some discomfort when a motion is passed. Rarely, slight bleeding may also occur during evacuation.

Second-degree Piles: They usually appear as pea-sized swellings outside the anus after a bowel motion has been passed. They are usually retained inside the anus and may bleed and cause discomfort during passing stool with some degree of itching.

Third-degree Piles: The swollen blood vessels are so enlarged that they remain outside the anus permanently. These are known as external piles, and are more troublesome. Soreness and persistent irritation are the common features.

4. Butter Milk: It is the home remedy of choice in piles. 100ml well mixed with a little bit of black pepper powder, and salt should be taken daily for a few months at least. Ayurveda stresses upon daily intake of butter milk by the piles patients.

5. *Hareetaki*, popularly known as *harad* is a good remedy for constipation. The decoction of the fruit peel of *harad* (Terminala Chebula) is taken 1 cupful with jaggery at bed-time.

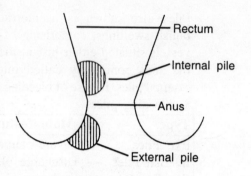

6. Rose petals, 11 in number crushed with 50 ml of water should be taken for 3 days on empty stomach. This is a very good remedy for bleeding piles. Banana fruit should not be taken for 1 year along with this treatment.

7. The decoction of sonth (dried ginger) is very useful in piles. It should be taken in the quantity of 30 to 50ml daily.

AYURVEDIC REMEDIES

1. *Triphalachurna*: This should be taken regularly to remove the constipation. 2 tsf of powder well mixed in a glass of lukewarm water should be taken orally before retiring to bed. Externally also it is widely used in different methods. One popular method is to take a plastic tub, fill it with warm water to a level where one can sit comfortably. Add 10 teaspoonfuls of *Triphalachurna* to the water and mix well for some time. Then the patient should sit in the tub, duly immersing the anus in the lukewarm water for 30 minutes. This should be carried out daily. This practice brings in enormous benefits to the piles patient.

2. *Abhayarista*: As an oral liquid preparation, it is also useful in constipation. 30 ml of the medicine dissolved in equal quantity of lukewarm water should be taken before going to bed.

3. *Arsha Harivati* is a common herbo-mineral compound prescribed by Ayurveda. 2 pills twice a day with some butter milk or warm water should be taken for 40 days. This gives great relief from piles.

4. *Arshony* tablet/ointment (Charak) 1-2 tablets thrice daily along with application of ointment before and after defecation.

5. Pilex tablet/ointment (Himalaya Drugs) are equally useful. Dosages are as above.
6. *Arshoghnivati* tablet (Baidyanath) 1 to 2 tablets with water or butter milk can be taken thrice or four times daily.
7. *Kankayan Vati* (Baidyanath) is equally good in both types of piles.
8. *Pileen, Arshon and Rasanjan Vati* tablets (Bhaat Ayurvedic Pharmacy) can cure both types of piles if taken in the dose of 1 to 2 tablets daily for 2 to 3 months.
9. *Kasisadi Tailam* when applied externally treats external piles completely.

For details on Ayurvedic Standard Medicines, refer to Glossary

11. DIARRHOEA

INTRODUCTION

Diarrhoea is defined as passage of loose, watery stools with increased frequency. When it is associated with vomiting with or without fever it is called *gastroenteritis*.

Causative Factors
Diarrhoea is common in all age-groups but children are more vulnerable. It is more common in poorly nourished children living in poor sanitary conditions. Most cases of diarrhoea are due to infection in the alimentary canal by viri, bacteria, parasites and fungi. Milk allergy and allergy to certain food substances can also give rise to diarrhoea. Certain medicines like antibiotics pain-killers and medicines for cancer can give rise to diarrhoea. Excessive, indigestible food substances and emotional factors can also give rise to diarrhoea.

TREATMENT

HOME REMEDIES

1. The decoction of *Dashmool* taken in the quantity of 20ml mixed with 2.5gms powder of *sonth* taken twice daily gives immediate relief.
2. The powder of *Harar* and *Pipal* taken in equal parts with warm water proves effective.
3. *Bel ki Giri* powder 2.5gms to 5gms taken twice or thrice a day is very useful in controlling diarrhoea.
4. The milk of goat boiled with equal quantity of water taken 20-50ml in divided doses gives relief in diarrhoea.

AYURVEDIC REMEDIES

1. *Kutaj Ghan Vati* is very useful in diarrhoea. It should be taken 1 tab three times a day.
2. Antidirol Forte (Bharat Ayurvedic Pharmacy) taken 1 tab three times a day controls diarrhoea in a single day.

3. Tab. Aurbimap (Maharishi Ayurved) is a very useful drug for viral and bacterial diarrhoea. The doses are 1 tab. 3 times a day.
4. *Sanjivini Vati* is also commonly used by Ayurvedic Physicians. It controls indigestion, flatulence and diarrhoea. The doses are 1 pill 2-3 times a day.
5. *Kutajarishta* 15ml mixed with equal quantity of water taken 2 times a day after meals.

DO'S & DON'TS

1. Any type of massages should be avoided.
2. Avoid greasy, spicy food and also overeating.
3. Any type of exercise should not be done.
4. Take light and appetising diet i.e., rice, ginger, *sonth, anar, jamum* etc.

12. DYSENTERY

INTRODUCTION

Dysentery refers to repeated passage of blood or mucus or both in the stool and invariably preceded by severe pain in the abdomen.

TREATMENT

HOME REMEDIES

1. *Bel* is very useful in dysentery. The soft pulp of fruit should be taken 1-2 tsf twice a day.
2. *Pipal* mixed with black pepper taken with milk controls dysentery.
3. Yoghurt taken 50gm mixed with small amount of honey taken 3 times a day controls dysentery.

AYURVEDIC REMEDIES

1. *Jati phaladivati* 1 tab. three times a day taken with *lassi* (butter milk) controls dysentery in early stage.
2. *Babularista* taken in a dose of 20ml mixed with 20ml of water given twice daily after meals.

Causative Factors

Dysentery is of two types—Amoebic dysentery due to Entamoeba histolytica, a parasite and Bacillary dysentery due to bacteria called Shigella. This disease is mainly due to consumption of water or food contaminated by these organisms.

Signs & Symptoms

The disease is characterized by passage of blood or mucus or both in stools. The frequency may vary from person to person. Invariably there is pain in the lower abdomen especially before passing stools. Appetite is poor and fever may be present. Patient feels very weak and restless.

3. *Dast bund* is a common drug used in dysentery and freely available in market. The doses are 1-2 tab. 3-4 times a day.

DO'S & DON'TS

Same as in the case of diarrhoea.

13. INTESTINAL WORMS

INTRODUCTION

The problem of infestation with intestinal worms is very common in Indian children. This is mainly due to lack of personal hygiene, poor sanitation and contamination of food and water. The different types of worms are roundworms, tapeworms, hookworms, threadworms and giardia.

TREATMENT

HOME REMEDIES

1. An apple a day keeps the worms away.
2. Tomatoes 2-3 in number with a pinch of black pepper and salt taken on empty stomach for 10 days prove very useful in worms.
3. Coconut water mixed with a small quantity of honey is very useful in worms.
4. *Ajwain* 5gm mixed with a pinch of salt taken on empty stomach for 5-7 days.

AYURVEDIC REMEDIES

1. *Krimi Mudgar Ras* — 1 pill 3 times a day.
2. *Krimi Kalanal Ras* — 1 pill 2 times a day for 7-10 days.
3. *Krimi Har Ras* 1 tab. daily for 10-15 days removes worms completely.

Causative Factors

The eggs of the worms find their way into the human body through contaminated food and water. Consumption of raw or improperly cooked vegetables and meat can give rise to growth and spread of worms. Drinking water from sources other than municipal taps without boiling, can also help in carrying cysts (eggs) of worms into the intestine.

Signs & Symptoms

The symptoms of the presence of worms vary according to their types. Some worms cause pain in the abdomen with either constipation or diarrhoea. Hookworms suck blood and give rise to anaemia. Roundworms are responsible for cough, vomiting, and loss of appetite. Urticaria, fever and bronchitis may also occur in some patients.

For details on Ayurvedic Standard Medicines, refer to Glossary

DO'S & DON'TS

1. Sweets should be avoided.
2. Sleeping during the days should be avoided.
3. Boiled water should be used especially during rainy season.
4. Fast food, junk foods are better avoided.

1. COMMON COLD

INTRODUCTION

Common cold, a routine complaint is of viral origin. It can be caused by any one of more than 200 viruses. Normally it is confined to the nose and throat although the virus can infect the larynx and lungs. It is communicable during the first 24 hours.

TREATMENT

There is no cure or prevention for cold. It is relieved naturally within a week. The cold is treated by attempting to relieve its symptoms such as headache, stuffy nose and congestion. Paracetamol tablets are generally taken to get relief from these symptoms.

HOME REMEDIES

These play a key role in the management of cold. These are:

Causative Factors

Cold can occur due to 200 or more viri. That is why we cannot take pills that would prevent colds by increasing immunity to the specific ones.

These viri are passed on in droplets when one coughs or sneezes.

Signs & Symptoms

These symptoms vary according to the virus involved. However general symptoms are:

- Sneezing
- Watery eyes
- Sore throat
- Cough and hoarseness
- Runny nose

In some individuals there may be unpleasant nasal discharge, headache and a slight temperature.

1. Black tea prepared with black pepper powder, dry ginger powder and *tulsi* leaves. This tea can be taken 3 to 4 times a day to get relief from runny nose, headache, and sore throat. It is as good as aspirin or paracetamol tablets.
2. Eat one *amla* twice a day. It is a rich source of vitamin C and strengthens the respiratory immunity.
3. Another simple home remedy is milk + turmeric. Add ½ tsp pure turmeric powder to a cup of hot milk, add some sugar and drink thrice a day to have relief. Inhalation of turmeric powder added to water and boiled is also a good remedy for cold.

AYURVEDIC REMEDIES

1. If *amla* is not available, its readymade preparation *Amlaki rasayan* in powder form is available in Ayurvedic stores. Take 3 gm of the powder along with warm milk twice a day.
2. *Luxmivilas Ras* (Nardia) is a drug of choice. It should be taken in the dose of 1 tablet thrice daily after meals with water.
3. Septilin tablet — one tab. twice daily.

For details on Ayurvedic Standard Medicines, refer to Glossary

DO'S & DON'TS

1. Chicken soup reduces the reproduction of viri that cause cold. If this is taken, cold may not be as intense.
2. Drink plenty of fluids like water, fruit juices, etc.
3. Most colds clear up on their own after one week, after which the infection spreads to the sinuses, ears, lungs etc., which is when you must consult your doctor.
4. Finally keep yourself warm and take plenty of rest.

DIETICS

Potatoes, brinjal, curd, and cold water should be avoided.

Supportive measures like hot fomentation, gentle massage and warm water baths should be practised to derive maximum benefit.

YOGA

Suitable yoga asanas in the condition are *shavasana* and *bhujangasana*.

2. COUGH

INTRODUCTION

In simple words cough is a reflex mechanism to expel any irritant from the trachea or wind pipe.

TREATMENT

HOME REMEDIES

Since most coughs are 'good' for the lungs it is desirable to allow the cough to run its normal course. Do not suppress a productive (wet) cough. Let the phlegm be expelled out.

1. Two gm of pure home made turmeric powder well mixed in a cup of warm milk, taken twice a day effectively checks the cough of bacterial origin. This should be continued for 15 days.
2. 5ml of fresh *tulsi* juice well mixed in 10ml of pure honey, chewed twice a day, calms down cough in children and adults.
3. In chronic coughs, crush 1 or 2 garlic cloves, add to a glass of milk, boil the milk till ½ glass of milk remains, then filter it, add little bit of sugar if desired, and make it into two parts. Take one part in the morning and another in the evening. Do it for a week. There will be remarkable improvement. However, acidity patients should not use it, since it may aggravate the acidity.
4. Similarly, onion juice can also be used. 5ml of fresh onion juice well mixed with 10ml of pure honey should be taken twice a day for 10 days.
5. Steam inhalation of turmeric in water is very good for controlling cough.

AYURVEDIC REMEDIES

1. *Sitopaladi Choorna*, a classical Ayurvedic preparation available in the stores, is the common drug. 3 to 5 gm of this powder, well mixed in 5ml of pure honey, should be taken twice or thrice a day. It works well for adults as well as children.
2. *Lavangadi Vati* — One tablet thrice a day should be chewed. It controls throat irritation and cough rapidly. One can carry this while travelling. Other products are listed separately in the glossary.

Causative Factors

Coughing can be due to number of conditions like colds and flu to more serious conditions like chronic bronchitis, asthma and whooping cough.

Signs & Symptoms

Generally coughs are worse in the morning and one may find that he/she is bringing up some thick yellow or green phlegm. Sometimes a minor irritation may start the cough reflex even though there is not sufficient material to clear from the lungs. This is known as a dry cough.

While coughing, if blood comes out or severe pain in the chest occurs, one should consult a doctor at once.

---

3. *Talicadi Churna* is also very useful in cough. The dose is 2.5 to 5gm twice daily with warm water.
4. *Kaph-ketu Ras* is another good preparation taken in the dose of 1 to 2 pills thrice daily with warm water.
5. Many cough syrups are available in the market which control cough. Of special mention are *Diakof* (Himalaya Drugs) and *Herbodil* (Dey's) which can be used by *diabetic* patients also.

For details on Ayurvedic Standard Medicines, refer to Glossary

DIET

One should avoid sour things like curd, lemon etc. and very cold water, soft drinks, and ice-creams. Meat should also be restricted.

3. WHOOPING COUGH

INTRODUCTION

Whooping cough is a bacterial infection of the respiratory system that usually affects children of 1-5 years. Being extremely contagious, the disease spreads quickly, often reaching epidemic levels. It can be fatal to small babies. Whooping cough can be successfully prevented by immunization in infancy in the form of 'Triple vaccine' DPT — diphtheria, tetanus and whooping cough.

TREATMENT

HOME REMEDIES

1. *Tulsi* leaves' juice (5ml) well mixed in 10 ml of pure honey should be given to the babies 3 to 4 times a day.
2. Garlic juice 3 to 4 times well mixed in 5 ml of pure honey can also be given thrice a day.

These measures give instant relief.

Causative Factors

Infection occurs from air borne bacteria called Bordetla pertussis, after close contact with the sufferer. The bacteria invade the nasal passage, respiratory tract and lungs, which produce a thick, sticky mucous discharge in an effort to combat the invasion.

Signs & Symptoms

The child first exhibits the signs of common cold. A cough develops with the characteristic 'whoop' sound as the lungs become congested. This can last from 2 to 10 weeks after exposure. Coughing episodes can occur up to 30 to 40 times a day which are violent and often lead to momentary loss of breath and vomiting. Babies who cannot cough up this mucous, are most at risk.

AYURVEDIC REMEDIES

1. *Talisadi Churna* 5gms + *Kapardika bhasma* 1gm should be given twice a day for 15 days.
2. Septilin (Himalaya Drugs) syrup 1 teaspoonful thrice daily for 2 weeks.
3. *Koflet* (Himalaya Drugs) syrup 1 teaspoonful thrice daily.
4. *Herbodil* (Himalaya Drugs) syrup 1 teaspoonful thrice daily mixed with 4 to 5 spoons of warm water.

For details on Ayurvedic Standard Medicines, refer to Glossary

4. FLU/INFLUENZA

INTRODUCTION

'Flu' is a viral infection of the upper respiratory tract. It is similar to common cold but happens to be more severe.

Signs & Symptoms

The typical symptoms include a sore throat, cough, fever, headache and aching muscles. The fever during flu is usually higher than in common cold. Similarly cough is also severe and lasts longer.

TREATMENT

HOME REMEDIES

1. *Tulsi* leaves in the form of infusion are highly effective or *Tulsi* leaves' juice can also be used in doses of 1 teaspoonful with 1 teaspoon of honey twice a day. This is a good remedy for 'flu' and cold. This can be taken as a preventive also when there is 'flu' in your city.
2. Similarly black pepper-dry ginger tea is also useful. This is generally prepared in Indian houses, during the prevalence of 'flu' and cold.
3. 1 tsp of pure turmeric powder or paste should be mixed in warm milk and can be taken 3 times a day.

AYURVEDIC REMEDIES

Those sold over the counter for 'flu' and common cold are:
1. *Trishun* Tablets: 1 tab. thrice a day with a cup of tea or warm water for 7 days is a sure remedy. It is a safe formulation.
2. *Trikatu Churna* is a cheaper version of *Trishun* available in the powder form. ½ tsp to 1 tsp with hot tea or water helps in checking the 'flu'.
3. *Tribhuvan Kirti Ras* is the drug of choice for flu in the dose of 1 to 2 tablets crushed and mixed with honey taken 3 to 4 times daily.

DO'S & DON'TS

1. Avoid heavy food, sour things including curd, exposure to cold wind and water.
2. Take light food like milk, bread, *kanji* etc.
3. Turmeric clears the lungs, relieves constipation and activates the liver thereby speeding up recovery. GARLIC is another useful home remedy.

5. SNEEZING

INTRODUCTION

Sneezing is a sudden and involuntary violent expiration preceded by inspiration. During sneezing, the mouth generally remains closed, so that the current of air is directed through the nose.

HOME REMEDIES

1. Take 2 drops of Badam Rogan (Hamdard) on palm, rub it and put it in both the nostrils and take a deep breath. It is very good in controlling sneezing.
2. Take 1 teaspoon of *besan* (gram flour), roast it with 1 teaspoon of pure ghee. Add a cup of milk and 4-5 *badams*. Boil it for 2-3 minutes. It should be taken at bed time. Water should not be taken after it.

Causative Factors

Sneezing normally occurs due to some irritation in the mucous membrane of the noses or the paranasal sinuses. It is commonly due to some allergic substances which may be eaten or inhaled. A cold draft of air or a cold humid weather precipitates sneezing. Dust, chemicals, smoke, pollen in the air can trigger sneezing. Eating certain food stuffs like ice-cream, cold drinks, banana, curd can induce sneezing attacks.

AYURVEDIC REMEDIES

1. *Luxmi Vilas Ras* (Nardia) is the drug of choice. 1 tab. three times a day.
2. Tab. Septilin (Himalaya Drugs Co.) 1-2 tab. 2-3 times a day.

DO'S & DON'TS

1. Patients should be kept warm.
2. Avoid direct heat or cold.
3. Patient should consume a lot of water and liquids.
4. *Shirodhara* is very effective in sneezing.

6. ASTHMA

INTRODUCTION

Asthma is one of the most prevalent health complaints. It is a condition wherein the patient has repeated attacks of wheezing, which usually clear up completely with medical treatment. Attacks produce a variety of disabilities from mild distress to severe incapacity.

Asthma can develop at any time in life but mostly starts in childhood.

ASTHMATIC TRIGGERS

1. First attack is usually set off by a lung infection.
2. Subsequent attacks are brought about by similar infections as even an ordinary cold.
3. Allergies. Drugs which the patient is allergic to may set off an attack.
4. Exercise.
5. Emotional trauma like anger, sorrow etc.
6. Sudden fluctuations in weather and temperature.

Causative Factors

- In asthmatics, the bronchial tube muscles which take air to the air-spaces in the lungs become narrow due to contraction, and air cannot move freely in or out of the lungs.
- Bronchial tubes also produce more mucous than usual thereby further reducing air movement.

Signs & Symptoms

- Wheezing is a characteristic symptom of asthma.
- Cough sometimes accompanies.
- Pulse rate rises.
- Inability to speak due to breathlessness.
- Typical difficulty in breathing out rather than breathing in.

TREATMENT

HOME REMEDIES

NOTE: Home remedies are found useful in mild attacks. However, in severe attacks, medical intervention or hospitalization may be necessary.

1. The juice of one clove of garlic (after removing the outer layer) is mixed with a tsp of honey and taken twice a day, to dilate the contracted bronchial tubes.

CAUTION: Patients of ulcers and bleeding disorders should abstain from the above remedy.

2. ½ tsp of *hing* (asafoetida) 50ml of sesame oil and a pinch of camphor are mixed and applied on the chest to relieve congestion and uneasiness.
3. 1 tsp full each of:
   (a) green ginger juice.
   (b) betel leaf juice, and

(c) juice of one clove of garlic

are mixed and taken thrice a day, 1 tsp each time.

4. Some camphor *(karpur)* and *hing* (asafoetida) are mixed well and pills of pea size are made. 1-2 pills taken with some hot water, 3 to 4 times a day, give relief.

5. *Tulsi* leaves' juice with honey is also beneficial. 1 tsp of *tulsi* juice & 1 tsp of honey should be taken 3 times a day.

6. Onion juice also can be taken similarly.

7. *Pipal, amla* and *sonth* are taken in equal quantities crushed in the form of churana and taken with honey, *mishri* (sugar candy) and *ghee* give good results in mild attacks.

8. *Gur* mixed with equal quantity of mustard oil taken for 21 days gives almost permanent relief.

9. The powder of *pipal* taken along with *sendha namak* (rock salt) and mixed with the juice of ginger gives results in 7 days.

AYURVEDIC REMEDIES

1. *Sitopaladi Choornam*: 5gm (1 tsp) of powder mixed with 2 tsp of honey, should be taken twice a day. (To be avoided by diabetics)

2. *Vasa Kantakari Lehyam*: 2 tsp of this semi-solid preparation may be taken followed by some warm milk.

3. *Dab-Dama*, liquid (Dabur) taken in the dose of 6 to 18 drops depending upon age and severity of disease along with water gives very good results.

4. *Chavanaprasa* is a rich source of vitamin C and is used as a tonic especially for bronchial asthma in a dose of 5-10gm with milk at bed time.

5. *Agastya rasayana* is usually given to people who are asthmatics with constipation, sneezing, blocking of nostrils and congestion of throat. Doses are same as above.

Care should be taken to see that the normal appetite is maintained.

For details on Ayurvedic Standard Medicines, refer to Glossary

DO'S & DON'TS

AVOID:

1. All Cold items : Ice cream, yoghurt, butter milk, cold drinks, lemon etc.

2. Allergy-triggering factors known to the patient.

3. Eggs, guava, cucumber.

4. Sleeping during the day.

5. Use garlic, *hing*, tea, warm water in plenty.

6. Take hot water bath only.

7. Protect the body with warm clothing in chilly weather.

7. SINUSITIS

INTRODUCTION

Sinusitis is the inflammatory condition of the mucous membrane lining the sinuses — the bone cavities leading from the nose. It usually follows a common cold, flu or other infections. Infecting germs sometimes enter the sinuses or chambers on either side of the nasal passage, causing sinus problems.

HOME REMEDIES

1. Garlic: The fresh juice of 3 to 4 garlic cloves, with 2 teaspoonfuls of honey, should be taken twice a day. It is a proven antibacterial, and analgesic.
2. Onion: Fresh juice of onion, well mixed in honey is also of great help in sinusitis.
3. Black pepper: 5gms of black pepper should be powdered finely, and this, well mixed in a cup of warm milk, if taken regularly, prevents recurrent attacks. It is a good anti-infective.
4. Steam inhalation is very good for sinusitis.

AYURVEDIC REMEDIES

1. *Maha Laxmi Vilas Ras* (SIRO) : 1 tablet twice a day with *Triphala quatha* is a good remedy for this painful condition.
2. *Chitraka Hareetaki* available in *lehya* form is a proven remedy. 2 teaspoons of this medicine should be mixed in a glass of warm milk, and taken twice a day.
3. Nasal inhalation of steam for 5 minutes gives good relief. A few drops of *Jeevandhara* (a mixture of camphor, menthol, etc.) should be added to the hot water, after which the steam should be inhaled twice a day.
4. Septilin (Himalaya Drugs) tablet 1 to 2 tablets twice daily for 4 to 6 weeks.
5. *Laxmi Vilas Ras* (Nardia) 1 tab. thrice daily for the same period.
6. *Shad Bindu Taila* can be used for inhalation 1 to 2 drops twice a day.

DO'S & DON'TS

DIET: Fried, refrigerated and starchy foods should be avoided. The patient should also avoid use of perfumes, scented oils etc.

For details on Ayurvedic Standard Medicines, refer to Glossary

Causative Factors

The sinuses generally contain nothing but air, but if there is a great deal of catarrh in the nose, the holes connecting the sinuses to it can get blocked and filled with mucous, which may then become infected. This is called 'sinusitis'.
Some people are more prone to sinusitis, than others. This is because they tend to get a lot of catarrh due to nasal allergy or it may be that the holes draining the sinuses are smaller than usual and so more liable to get blocked. Chronic rhinitis or a cold may bring on sinusitis.

Signs & Symptoms

Excessive or constant sneezing, a running nose, blockage of one or both nostrils, headaches and pressure around the head, eyes and face are experienced. The face is very tender to touch, but not usually swollen.

8. BRONCHITIS

INTRODUCTION

Bronchitis is characterized by the inflammation of the bronchi of the lungs which result in the discharge of a muco-purulent substance known as phlegm or sputum.

TREATMENT

HOME REMEDIES

1. The juice of ginger 1 teaspoonful mixed with honey taken thrice a day proves effective in Bronchitis.
2. The decoction of *tulsi*, ginger, black pepper in equal quantities taken 20-25ml three times a day.
3. *Mulathi* chewed over a period of few hours gives relief.
4. *Jushanda* is a popular remedy for Bronchitis. Take 1 teaspoon of this powder, add to it a cup of water. Boil it till half of it remains. Add some sugar or honey and take it at bed time and in the morning before breakfast.

AYRVEDIC REMEDIES

1. *Talisadi Churna* taken ½ to 1 teaspoon along with honey and ginger juice gives relief in a day or two. The doses can be taken three times a day.
2. *Khadiravati* should be kept in mouth and sucked slowly. This gives relief in bronchitis associated with congested throat. 4-6 pills can be sucked over a day.
3. *Vasarishta* is a liquid taken 15ml + 15ml. of water twice a day after meals.
4. *Haridara Khand* 5gm of it mixed with a cup of warm milk at bed time proves effective.

For details on Ayurvedic Standard Medicines, refer to Glossary

Causative Factors

This disease is mainly seen in cigarette smokers. Smoking induces inflammation of the airway with obstruction of the bronchi. Dust and air pollution also contribute largely to this disease. This disease is more common during winter months but when chronic it may be present all the year around.

Signs & Symptoms

- Severe cough especially during the mornings of winter months.
- Cough is productive (contains sputum) in nature.
- Sputum may be scanty, mucoid, thick with occasional streaks of blood. Yellow sputum indicates infection.
- Patient may complain of tightness around the chest.
- Breathlessness on exertion may be reported.
- Wheezing or whistling sound may be heard while breathing.
- Fever when infection is present.

DO'S & DON'TS

1. Steam inhalation is very good.
2. Curd and sour things should be avoided.
3. Sour fruits including banana and guava are also contraindicated.
4. Exposure to cold wind and rain should be avoided.

9. PLEURISY

INTRODUCTION

The inflammation of the pleura which is the membrane covering the lungs is known as pleurisy. This is of three types. If associated with a lot of fluid it is called pleural effusion and when pus is formed inside it is called purulent effusion or empyema. When the inflammation persists for a long time and fibrin is deposited, it is called dry pleurisy.

Causative Factors

The causes are numerous. They are:
1. Tuberculosis, 2. Pneumonia, 3. Heart failure, 4. Liver and pancreatic diseases, 5. Cancer, 6. Hypothyroidism.

Signs & Symptoms

● Pain in the chest.
● Cough.
● Difficulty in breathing.
● Difficulty in lying down.
● Fever.

TREATMENT

HOME REMEDIES

1. Garlic clove 1 in number taken on empty stomach with water is good.
2. Decoction prepared with *tulsi* leaves, *pudina, lavang,* black pepper proves useful, 50ml 2-3 times a day.
3. *Triphala Churna* ½ teaspoon twice daily is good if patient is constipated.
4. Bed rest is good for these type of patients.

AYURVEDIC REMEDIES

1. *Shringa Bhasma* is the drug of choice. Half gram of this is to be given to patient 3-4 times a day mixed with honey.
2. *Ras Sindoora* and *Suvarna Vasantha Malni Rasa* are other Ayurvedic medicines but these should be taken under supervision.

For details on Ayurvedic Standard Medicines, refer to Glossary

DO'S & DON'TS

1. Fried and refrigerated food stuff is strictly prohibited.
2. Physical exercises, sexual indulgence, exposure to cold wind and rain should be refrained.
3. Patient should not sleep during day time.

10. TUBERCULOSIS

INTRODUCTION

This is a very common disease seen in India and other developing countries. It primarily affects the lung through the bones, lymph nodes, intestine. Brain and other organs may also be affected.

TREATMENT

HOME REMEDIES

1. Garlic (Lahsuna) is a very useful home remedy. Thirty grains of garlic are to be boiled with 150 ml. of milk + 50ml of water. When about 50ml remains, it should be filtered and twice given to patient.
2. The powder of amla should be given to patient in a dose of ½ teaspoon daily with water, one hour before meals or after meals.
3. Pippali (*piper longum*) is also very effective. One teaspoonful powder of it can be given three times a day mixed with honey.

AYURVEDIC REMEDIES

1. *Chavanprasa* is a drug of choice. It can be given to any type of tuberculosis patient 5gm to 10gm twice daily with milk.
2. *Drakhsasava* 15-20ml with 15-20ml of water twice daily after meals.
3. *Vasa-avleham/vasa-rishta* is also very useful.
4. *Mahalaxmi Vilas Rasa* is also commonly used by physicians. It should be taken under supervision as it contains gold.

Causative Factors

This disease is caused by bacteria called Mycobacterium tuberculosis. The infection is spread by patients of tuberculosis who discharge these bacteria in their sputum or nasal secretions during bouts of coughing or sneezing. Malnutrition can reduce the immunity of the individual and predispose him to this infection. People living in crowded areas with inadequate ventilation and sunshine are at high risk.

Signs & Symptoms

- Continuous cough over prolonged periods
- Pain in the chest
- Fever
- Coughing out blood
- Lethargy
- Weight loss

DO'S & DON'TS

1. All dry fruits especially grapes and almond oil are useful.
2. Milk and eggs should be given.
3. Curd and other sour things as banana, guava are best avoided.
4. Cow's milk and its products are useful.
5. Patient should take physical or mental rest.

1. BLEEDING NOSE

INTRODUCTION

'Epistaxis' is the medical term for bleeding from the nose.

TREATMENT

HOME REMEDIES

1. The patient should wash his face and head with cold water.
2. Icepacks should be applied from outside on the nose.
3. One should not sneeze or put any type of strain on the nose which aggravates bleeding.
4. If B.P. is high, anti-hypertensives should be taken under medical advice.
5. Juice of flower of pomegranate should be used for deep inhalation.
6. Juice of Durva grass 5 to 10 drops in each nostril gives immediate relief.

Causative Factors

The most common cause of epistaxis in young people is not known unless it is a result of picking of the nose or injury. In summer these episodes occur more in young persons. In older patients, rarely high blood pressure can cause epistaxis, especially if the diastolic pressure is more than 110 mm/Hg. High exposure to heat sources such as the sun or fire also leads to bleeding.

AYURVEDIC REMEDIES

1. *Vasa Avalehya* is a semisolid sweet preparation. One teaspoonful well mixed in a cup of cold milk should be taken orally 3 times a day. It checks the bleeding. Inspite of all these measures, if bleeding does not stop, an ENT surgeon's consultation is a must without delay.
2. *Anu Tailam* in a dose of 2 to 5 drops in each nostril for inhalation can stop bleeding.
3. Styplon tablet (Himalaya Drugs) 1 to 2 tablets twice or thrice daily gives very good results.
4. *Chavanaprash* can be given one teaspoon twice daily with milk. It is a rich source of Vitamin C.
5. *Amla Churan* is also helpful in such conditions in the dose of ½ teaspoon twice daily with water.

DO'S & DON'TS

The patient or person, who has a history of bleeding should avoid all hot and spicy things in eatables. He should maintain normal blood-pressure. He should not remain awake at nights.

2. SORE TONGUE

INTRODUCTION

Sore tongue medically known as stomatitis is a very common symptom. Most of the doctors routinely prescribe B-complex tablets, terming it B-complex deficiency. In fact in many instances it is not so.

Causative Factors

The most common reason of sore tongue where is tongue is red and bald is 'Antibiotic glossitis'. Indiscriminate use of antibiotics causes (1) Disturbances to normal bacterial flora and over growth of fungus (2) B-complex deficiency and lastly (3) Chemical irritation of tongue. Out of these factors, B-complex deficiency is the least important cause.

Some people get attacks of sore mouth or tongue very often. During the episode, ulcers appear on the tongue or buccal mucous membrane. They are very painful, look yellowish and are surrounded by a red margin. They may have varying appearances too. The important point is that these appear for no reason and disappear within a week or ten days. These can be termed as 'stress ulcers'. They are not harmful to the body, but are only of nuisance value.

| TREATMENT |

HOME REMEDIES

TURMERIC POWDER which is powdered at home is a highly useful healing agent in this condition. ½ teaspoonful of turmeric powder well mixed in a cup of warm milk along with some sugar should be consumed twice a day.

'ALUM' is highly useful in this condition. Some quantity of alum is fried over a frying pan by which it gets dehydrated and swollen. The colour changes to whitish. This should be powdered and mixed well with honey and applied over the affected areas.

AYURVEDIC REMEDIES

Before application of this, 2 tsf of *Triphalachurna* mixed in warm water is used to rinse the sore mouth. A popular Ayurvedic remedy available over the counter for this 'sore tongue' is *Khadiradi Vati* tablets. These should be chewed 3 to 4 times a day. This drug heals the oral ulcers quickly. One of the important ingredients of this preparation is *Kattha* used in *pan* — a domestically available item.

For details on Ayurvedic Standard Medicines, refer to Glossary

One should discontinue alcohol taking and excessive tea drinking, betel nut/ clove chewing etc.

43

3. HOARSE VOICE/ LARYNGITIS

INTRODUCTION

Laryngitis is the term used to denote the inflammatory condition of the larynx — the voice box.

TREATMENT

GENERAL: The hoarseness and irritation may last for up to a week and can be relieved by resting the voice and stopping smoking.

HOME REMEDIES

1. Inhalation: Inhale the vapours coming out of hot water in which a few drops of eucalyptus oil have been added, for about 10 minutes.
2. Add some black pepper powder to a cup of warm milk, and drink the mixture twice a day. A little bit of sugar can also be added, if desired.
3. The fresh juice of *tulsi* leaves (½ tsf) and 1 tsp of honey well mixed, should be taken 3 to 4 times a day.
4. *Akkarakara* (root of Anacyclus pyrethrum). Make a fine powder of *Akkarakara,* and use in small doses of 300 to 600mg twice a day with warm water. This increases the secretion of saliva, and is thereby useful in hoarse voice.
5. Steam inhalation of turmeric water. Add a pinch of turmeric powder *(haldi)* to 15 to 20ml of water.

Causative Factors

- Acute laryngitis is a short-term viral or bacterial throat infection, often caused due to an attack of cold.
- It may also be caused by some other irritants, like smoking, *pan* chewing, *gutkha*, alcohol etc.
- Some people are prone to chronic laryngitis, such as heavy smokers, and those who work in a dusty environment or who use their voices continuously like singers, speakers etc.

Signs & Symptoms

- The characteristic sign is a hoarse voice, which may lead to total voice loss.
- A sore throat and difficulty in swallowing are also common.
- Chronic laryngitis develops over a period of time and sufferers may cough and clear their throats regularly and always have a hoarse voice.

AYURVEDIC REMEDIES

1. *Talisadi Churna* is a powdered drug useful in this condition. 3 gms of this powder, well mixed in honey or lukewarm water can be taken 3 to 4 times a day.

2. *Lavangadivati*: These pills are specially prescribed in throat diseases. 1 to 2 pills can be chewed 3 to 4 times a day. It is a good remedy for laryngitis.
3. *Yasti Madhu* is also a useful remedy. 2gms of powder well mixed in a cup of milk should be taken twice a day.
4. *Septilin Tablet* (Himalaya Drugs) 1 to 2 tablets twice daily for 4 to 6 weeks.
5. *Kaph-ketu Ras* 1 to 2 pills thrice daily for 4 weeks.

For details on Ayurvedic Standard Medicines, refer to Glossary

DIET

All irritating food stuffs like pickles and spices, should be avoided. Cold water, curd, smoking, and alcohol are also to be avoided for better results.

4. PUS IN THE EAR

INTRODUCTION

Pus in the ear occurs due to inflammation of the ear which is caused by certain bacteria and viruses.

HOME REMEDIES

Garlic, onion and ginger are useful both externally and internally.

AYURVEDIC REMEDIES

1. *Laxmi Vilas Ras* (Nardia) is the drug of choice. One pill three times a day after meals with honey.
2. *Nirgundayadi Tail* is effective when used externally. One or two drops should be put into ear twice daily.
3. Septilin (Himalaya) 1-2 tabs twice daily for 15 days.

For details on Ayurvedic Standard Medicines, refer to Glossary

DO'S & DON'TS

The patient should not take bath nor should he expose himself to cold wind and rain.

Causative Factors

The organisms causing pus in the ear occur due to cough, cold and sinusitis. Initially running nose, cold or cough may be present but later the bacteria enter into the middle ear through the eustachian tube. In children the eustachian tube (connecting the throat and middle ear) is very short and hence infection of the ear is very common after an attack of cold, cough or sinusitis.

Signs & Symptoms

- When pus is formed in the middle ear, child complains of severe pain in the ear which is unbearable.
- In most cases the pus enters into the external ear and outside after the eardrum is ruptured. This reduces the earache and foul-smelling pus come out.
- Fever may be present in many cases.
- Vomiting, poor appetite, cough may be associated.

5. MOUTH ULCERS/ STOMATITIS

INTRODUCTION

Stomatitis refers to the inflammation of the mouth resulting in diffuse redness, blisters, ulcers and sulmucosal haemorrhages. The inner sides of the cheeks, tongue, floor of the tongue and palate may be affected.

TREATMENT

HOME REMEDIES

1. Constipation is the root cause. It should be avoided by taking *Triphala Churna* 1 teaspoonful at bed time.
2. Gargles can be done with its decoction mixed with honey.
3. Neem is also very useful in toothpaste form or in tooth powder form.

AYURVEDIC REMEDIES

1. *Khadiradivati* is the drug of choice, 1-2 pills chewed or taken with water three times a day.
2. *Irimedadi Taila* is also very effective for external use.

For details on Ayurvedic Standard Medicines, refer to Glossary

DO'S & DON'TS

1. One should avoid tobacco in any form.
2. Use toothpaste or toothpowder regularly twice daily.
3. Use of green vegetables and fruits should be encouraged.

Causative Factors

Ulcers may be caused by different types of organisms bacteria (syphilis) fungi (candidiasis) or viri (herpes simples). They may be due to toxicity of drugs and heavy metals. Nutritional dificiency (B Complex) may also be responsible. It may also be a sign of underlying diseases of the gastrointestinal system, skin, AIDS or even cancer.

Signs & Symptoms

These vary according to the cause. Pain and difficulty in swallowing is present in all cases. Some may complain of fever and foul-smelling odour from the mouth.

6. BAD BREATH

INTRODUCTION

It is a harmless condition known as 'Halitosis' in medical parlance.

TREATMENT

HOME REMEDIES

1. Clean teeth regularly with neem paste.
2. Wash mouth with a tsf of *Triphalachurna* or neem bark powder dissolved in warm water 3 to 4 times a day.
3. *Chhoti Elaichi* (green cardamom) is an excellent mouth freshener.
4. The decoction of *dhania* (coriander) can be used as mouthwash.
5. The gargles of cold decoction of aloe vera mixed with honey is very effective in chronic bad breath.

Causative Factors

Halitosis is caused usually due to poor care of teeth and gums. Eating strongly flavoured food, such as garlic or onions, can also cause it. Chronic constipation, respiratory infections, or very bad sinusitis may also cause bad breath.

Signs & Symptoms

Strong and unpleasantly odoured breath.

AYURVEDIC REMEDIES

1. Above all to keep the bowels free and to remove constipation, using *Deendayal Churna* 5gms mixed in warm water daily at bed time is helpful. This checks acidity, constipation and gases and keeps the entire digestive system from mouth to anus clean, thereby controlling bad breath.
2. *Eladivati* pills and other digestives can be chewed 3 to 4 times a day or as and when bad breath is noticed. These pills when sucked, immediately control bad breath and if even after all these measures, bad breath persists, consulting a dentist is judicious.
3. *Larangadi Vati* can be chewed 4 to 5 times daily for controlling bad breath.
4. Gum-Tone tooth powder (Charak) used twice daily for 15 days gives very good results.
5. *Irimadadi Tailam* can be massaged on the gums to avoid bad breath.
6. *Khadivadi Vati* chewed or swallowed orally treats all the diseases of the mouth and oral cavity.
7. *Kanth Sudhar Vati* can be chewed upto 10 times a day for controlling bad breath.
8. *Mastan* tablet (Zandu) is very effective in controlling bad breath immediately.
9. *Tambool Ranjan* (Zandu) is a digestive tonic used for curing poor appetite, bad breath and toothache.

For details on Ayurvedic Standard Medicines, refer to Glossary

7. PYORRHOEA

INTRODUCTION

Pyorrhoea is characterized by copious discharge of pus from the root of the teeth and gums.

TREATMENT

HOME REMEDIES

1. Prop-root of banyan tree should be used for brushing teeth.
2. Twigs or tender branches of neem can also be used for same purpose.

AYURVEDIC REMEDIES

1. 'Gum tone' (Charak) powder used daily for 2 months gives good results.
2. *Triphala* powder or decoction of it is very useful if patient is constipated.
3. *Bakula* and *Babula* are very good and are used as tooth powders.
4. *Dasana Samskara Churna* is another drug of choice. This is either used by finger or soft brush daily for 15 days.

For details on Ayurvedic Standard Medicines, refer to Glossary

DO'S & DON'TS

1. Food rich in Vitamin-C is good for these type of patients.
2. Vegetables like *karela*, potato and drumstick are useful.
3. Avoid things which stick to the roots of teeth as far as possible.

Causative Factors

Poor oral hygiene is the main cause of pyorrhoea. Not brushing the teeth daily and not cleaning the mouth after intake of food give rise to infection by various types of organisms.

Signs & Symptoms

The patient has difficulty in chewing food especially hard ingredients since these produce pain and bleeding from the gums. Pus from the gums and teeth produces foul smell in the mouth and teeth fall out one by one. Some may have fever if infection is severe or diarrhoea and gastritis due to swallowing of pus.

8. TOOTH-ACHE

INTRODUCTION

Good teeth are the indication of good health, but often these are prone to infections, as these are overused and exposed to a variety of food and drinks. Toothache is a most common complaint.

TREATMENT

HOME REMEDIES

Apply a hot water bag or ice bag to the side of the face — whichever gives most relief.

1. Clove Oil is the standard home remedy. A few drops should be applied twice or thrice a day with the help of sterilized cotton swabs.
2. An antiseptic lotion for gargling can also be used as required. This can be prepared by mixing 5ml each of clove oil and eucalyptus oil, some menthol and sufficient water.
3. Garlic is an effective home remedy for toothache. A paste prepared from one or two garlic cloves and a little bit of salt should be applied on the affected tooth. Garlic is a good pain-killer, anti-inflammatory and anti-bacterial agent.
4. Onion also contains the above properties, and a small piece of onion can be placed in the affected area.

Causative Factors

The chief cause of tooth-ache is decay of teeth, resulting from bad eating habits like over-indulgence in sweets, ice creams, soft drinks, sour things and sugar items. Bacteria present in the mouth cavity break sugar down into acids, which interact with the calcium in the enamel to cause decay or erosion.

Signs & Symptoms

Tooth-ache may be constant throughout the day and night or it may occur now and then for a short period depending on the degree of dental damage. The character of the pain may be dull, sharp, shooting or radiating towards ears, and head. Severe headache may also follow.

AYURVEDIC REMEDIES

1. *Triphala Churna* — 10 grams of the powder should be soaked in a glass full of hot water for some time. Once this solution becomes lukewarm it should be used for gargling purpose. If used regularly, it not only reduces the pain but also prevents further decay of teeth.
2. *Kanchanara Guggul*, in doses of 2 pills twice a day, gives relief from inflammation.
3. 'Gum tone' tooth powder, if used regularly, prevents dental problems.
4. *Irimedadi Taila* is the specific Ayurvedic remedy for dental problems. This should be applied externally on the affected teeth.

For details on Ayurvedic Standard Medicines, refer to Glossary

DIET

The items enumerated as causative factors above, should be avoided.

9. TONSILLITIS

INTRODUCTION

Tonsillitis is an inflammatory condition of the tonsils which lie one on each side of the throat. This inflammation occurs due to infection. It is a common childhood problem.

TREATMENT

HOME REMEDIES

1. Garlic paint: Make a paste of garlic cloves, smear it on a piece of cotton wool, warm it on a low flame and squeeze the juice. Add equal quantity of honey and swab the inflamed tonsils with this juice for prompt relief.
2. Milk + Turmeric: A glass of warm milk, well mixed with a pinch of pure turmeric powder and black pepper powder is taken twice a day for 10 days.

AYURVEDIC REMEDIES

1. *Kanchanara Guggul* 2 pills twice a day with warm water.
2. Septillin tablets 1 tab. thrice a day.
3. *Kaph Ketu Ras* 2 tab. 3 times a day.
4. *Tundikeri Ras* 1 tab. 3 times a day.

For details on Ayurvedic Standard Medicines, refer to Glossary

---

Causative Factors

Tonsils are present to protect the upper respiratory tract from infection by trapping and destroying micro-organisms. In the process, sometimes they too become infected by the micro organisms.

Tonsillitis is common in children under ten years of age, although it occasionally occurs in young adults. When it occurs in adulthood, the symptoms are usually more severe.

Signs & Symptoms

The throat becomes sore and inflamed and there is often difficulty in swallowing. Fever, headache, earache and swollen neck glands are other possible symptoms & signs. If symptoms persist for more than 24 hours or if there is pus visible on the tonsils, consulting an ENT specialist is essential.

1. CATARACT

INTRODUCTION

Opacification of the lens of the eye or its capsule (covering) sufficient to interfere with vision is called cataract.

TREATMENT

HOME REMEDIES

1. The eyes should be washed daily with *Triphala* water. 1 teaspoonful of powder should be added to a glass of water at night. It is filtered in the morning and is ready for use.

AYURVEDIC REMEDIES

1. *Maha Triphala Ghritam* is popularly used in early stage of cataract. The doses are two teaspoonfuls twice daily with a cup of milk one hour before taking food.
2. *Chandrodaya Vati* is used for external use. It is rubbed over a clean stone with water, and the paste is applied in the eye.

Causative Factors

Cataract may be caused due to following factors:
- Malnutrition
- Vitamin A or B deficiency
- High myopia (short-sight)
- Diabetes
- Old age
- Infections of the eye

Signs & Symptoms

Initially patient complains of blurring of vision in the early stages of the disease. Later when the cataract matures, complete vision is impaired in the affected eye. If treatment is not done, the cataract becomes hypermature and leads to increase in intra-ocular pressure (glaucoma).

OTHER MEASURES

Exposure to excessive heat or sun is prohibited. If the cataract is fully matured, then surgery is the only treatment

2. MYOPIA/SHORT SIGHT

INTRODUCTION

Myopia or short-sight refers to difficulty in seeing objects at a distance.

Causative Factors

Due to the change in the curvature of the refracting surface of the eye or abnormal refractivity of the media of the eye, myopia results. This gives rise to parallel rays transmitted by the objects focussing in front of the retina. The problem is solved by wearing spectacles with concave lens of appropriate curvature. Malnutrition, vitamin deficiency, improper reading habits, prolonged viewing of television or working on computers can lead to myopia.

TREATMENT

HOME REMEDIES

1. *Triphala* powder is a good remedy. It can be used externally as well as internally. The usages are same as in cataract.

AYURVEDIC REMEDIES

1. *Yasti Madhu* is the drug of choice for this condition. The powder of this is used one teaspoonful mixed with one teaspoonful of honey and ½ teaspoonful of pure ghee daily on empty stomach twice daily.
2. *Shadbindu Taila* is also good for it. 1-2 drops of it should be put in each nostril and deeply inhaled once in the morning.

DO'S & DON'TS

1. Constipation and nasal congestion should be avoided.
2. Fried and spicy things are to be avoided.
3. Cow's ghee should be taken with food.
4. Strain of eyes should be avoided.

3. STYE

INTRODUCTION

Stye refers to the inflammation and infection of the eyelid. It may affect the skin of eyebrows or the eyelid, more commonly the lower eyelid.

TREATMENT

HOME REMEDIES

Same as before (as in Cataract Myopia).

AYURVEDIC REMEDIES

Chandrodaya Vati is the drug of choice for external use. But it should be used under supervision.

DO'S & DON'TS

1. The patients should avoid all sour foods and drinks.
2. Curds are specially prohibited.
3. Reading is not advisable.
4. Patient should not be awake till late hours at nights.

Causative Factors

It is usually caused by certain pus-forming bacteria called the staphylococci. It is due to lack of regular cleaning and washing of the eyes. Poor health, malnutrition, conjunctivitis and infections of the eyelids can give rise to stye formation.

Signs & Symptoms

Stye causes pain and uneasiness. Sometimes fever may be present. Difficulty in vision is sometimes present. After 4 to 5 days the redness gives rise to pus formation and once the pus comes out, the patient is relieved of pain. Styes may be recurrent in nature.

---

4. CONJUNCTIVITIS

INTRODUCTION

The 'sclera' or 'white' of the eye is covered by transparent membrane known as the 'conjunctiva' which easily becomes inflamed if exposed to irritation or infection. This inflammation is known as 'conjunctivitis'. Normally the white part of the eyeball appears pinkish or reddish in colour.

TREATMENT

HOME REMEDIES

Fresh breastmilk is the best home remedy for conjunctivitis. It should be poured into both eyes 4 to 5 times daily.

Causative Factors

- More often, conjunctivitis is caused by an allergy to pollen, house dust, or make-up — this type is known as allergic conjunctivitis.
- Reaction to chemical irritants like factory fumes, tobacco smoke or excessive chlorine in swimming pool water, is known as chemical conjunctivitis.
- Allergic and chemical conjunctivitis are not contagious. However conjunctivitis caused by bacteria or viral infections are communicable from one person to another rapidly. Therefore this type is known as infectious conjunctivitis. Strict hygienic practices are

Contd ...

AYURVEDIC REMEDIES

A doctor must be consulted first, before using any of the remedies.

1. *Triphala Lotion:* 15 grams of fresh *Triphalachurna* should be soaked in one glass (200ml) of pure water for ½ hour. Then boil it on mild flame till ¼ volume remains. Filter it through a clean cloth. Use this lotion for washing the affected eyes 3 to 4 times a day. This clears the eyes.

2. *Triphala Churna* can be taken internally also in the condition. 5 grams of powder with water twice a day in viral type is very useful.

3. *Amla* (Indian gooseberry): The freshly extracted juice in the dose of 2 teaspoonful thrice a day is rewarding.

   a. I-Tone (Dey's) eye drops should be put into both the eyes, 4 to 5 times in a day.

   b. Optho Care (Himalaya Drug Co.) eye drops is also an effective remedy for conjunctivitis. 4 to 6 drops should be put in the eyes.

For details on Ayurvedic Standard Medicines, refer to Glossary

DO'S & DON'TS

1. Wear dark glasses.
2. Wear goggles while swimming.
3. Do not touch your eyes unnecessarily.
4. Do not share towels, etc.

essential, otherwise it may become an epidemic.

Signs & Symptoms

Red, itchy, burning eyes with watering inflammation over inner eyelids is the main feature along with sticky discharge from eyes, which seals the lids together overnight.

In bacterial type, the discharge appears like pus and if viral in nature, the discharge will be thinner and more watery.

V. DISEASES OF THE HEART & CIRCULATORY SYSTEM

1. HEART DISEASE

INTRODUCTION

Heart disease refers to a clinical syndrome characterized by chest pain produced by increased work by the heart. It is caused by obstruction of the coronary arteries mainly by deposition of fat. A reduction in the flow of blood leads to chest pain and heart attack or angina.

Causative Factors

Certain risk factors important for causing coronary heart disease are as follows:

1. Excessive smoking, 2. Hypertension, 3. Increased blood cholesterol levels, 4. Diabetes, 5. Lack of exercise, 6. Obesity, 7. Excessive alcohol consumption, 8. Mental stress.

Signs & Symptoms

- Pain in front of chest either on the left, centre or even on the right side. Pain is increased by physical activity. Intermittent pain.
- Pain may spread to the arms, neck, jaws and even upper part of abdomen.
- Difficulty in breathing is present in most acute cases and in some chronic cases.
- Sweating is seen in acute attacks.
- Irregular heart beat may be seen in some cases.

TREATMENT

HOME REMEDIES

1. One clove of garlic should be taken daily once on empty stomach.
2. Lots of fluids should be taken.
3. The decoction of *sonth* should be taken twice daily (30-50ml).
4. The decoction of bark of *neem* is also very good for heart diseases.

AYURVEDIC REMEDIES

1. *Arjunarishta* is a drug of choice. 15-20ml mixed with equal quantity of water twice daily after meals.
2. Tab *Abana* (Himalaya Drugs) 1-2 tab. twice daily acts as a cardioprotective.
3. Tab *Arjunin* (Charak) also checks heart diseases especially palpitation etc. Dose is 1-2 pills twice daily.
4. *Jawahar Mohrapisti* 120mg taken with *khamira* twice daily with milk.

DO'S & DON'TS

1. Rest during the day is a must.
2. Bowels should move regularly.
3. Morning walks are good.
4. Stimulants like tea, coffee and alcoholic drinks are very harmful for heart patients.

2. HYPERTENSION (HIGH BLOOD PRESSURE)

INTRODUCTION

Hypertension refers to an increase in the blood pressure of an individual depending on his age, sex, physical and mental activities, family history and diet.

TREATMENT

HOME REMEDIES

1. Garlic is an excellent drug. It is made to paste and taken with buttermilk.
2. Almond oil one teaspoonful at bed time with a cup of milk.
3. Diet should be salt restricted.

AYURVEDIC REMEDIES

1. *Sarpagandha* is used commonly for high blood pressure. 1 tab twice a day.
2. *Abana* 1-2 tab. twice daily for 6 weeks.
3. *Dhara* therapy is considered good. It should be done with medicated oil boiled with Bala and milk.
4. Tab *Shanta* (Bharat Ayurvedic Pharmacy) 1 tab. twice daily.

Causative Factors

In more than 95% of cases no specific underlying cause can be found. Such patients are said to have essential hypertension. In some cases hypertension may be secondary to some disease or abnormality leading to secondary hypertension. These causes are as follows:

- Excessive alcohol consumption.
- Pregnancy.
- Diseases of the kidneys.
- Hormonal disorders.
- Various drugs e.g. contraceptive pills, steroids, pain-killers etc.
- Other factors-excessive salt intake, lack of exercise and mental tension.

Signs & Symptoms

- Headache.
- Giddiness.
- Palpitation.
- Lack of sleep.
- Breathlessness on exertion.
- Easy fatigability.

For details on Ayurvedic Standard Medicines, refer to Glossary

DO'S & DON'TS

1. Hydrogenated oils should be avoided.
2. The patient should take such vegetables which help him keep his bowels clear.
3. Mental stress should be avoided.
4. Meditation is very effective for these type of patients.
5. *Palak*, a vegetable, should be avoided as far as possible, as it is rich in sodium element.
6. Salt should be restricted.

3. SWELLING OF THE BODY/OEDEMA

INTRODUCTION

Oedema refers to non-inflammatory swelling of the body. The swelling may be sometimes localized to the face, legs or abdomen and at times appears throughout the body.

Causative Factors

- Diseases of the heart.
- Diseases of the kidney.
- Liver diseases.
- Anemia.
- Malnutrition.
- Medicines—steroids, painkillers, hormones, antihypertensives.

Signs & Symptoms

These depend on the cause of oedema.

TREATMENT

HOME REMEDIES

1. *Gomutra* (cow's urine) is very good for massage on the affected par
2. Castor oil 10-15ml should be taken twice daily mixed with a cup of warm milk.
3. The powder of pepper mixed with the juice of *bel* leaves taken ½ teaspoonful two-three times a day.
4. The paste of lotus flower ½ teaspoonful mixed with milk taken twice daily for 15 days cures oedema completely.

AYURVEDIC REMEDIES

1. *Punarnava Mandoor* is commonly used for oedema 1 tab. three times a day after meals with water for about a month.
2. *Punarnava Guggulu* is another drug of choice 1-2 pills 2-3 times a day.

DO'S & DON'TS

1. Salt, fried items and curd are prohibited.
2. Ripe papaya should be taken on regular basis.
3. Patient should not sleep during day.
4. Excess of fat of any origin should be avoided.

4. ATHEROSCLEROSIS

INTRODUCTION

Atherosclerosis, popularly known as AS, denotes hardening of the arteries. This condition gradually builds up due to fatty deposits known as cholesterol and minerals collected in the walls of the arteries and render them less elastic and narrower. Because of this decrease in arterial diameter, blood flow is reduced, and gradually cuts off the supply of blood to heart, brain, muscles or kidneys.

THE MAJOR KILLER

1. Atherosclerosis is responsible for more deaths than any other cause.
2. 1/3 of deaths occur due to it.
3. Heart-attacks, strokes, and cramps develop because of the hardening and narrowing of the major arteries.

PREVENTION

This can be prevented, if all the causative factors, stated above are removed.

TREATMENT

Once atherosclerosis is suspected, the diagnosis can be confirmed by further investigations. Treatment has to be taken under expert medical supervision.

Causative Factors

Overeating of high animal-fat diet and refined sugar can lead to the hardening of arteries. Lack of exercise or physical activity, high cholesterol levels in the blood and cigarette smoking make the artery walls more permeable so that they are more likely to build up cholesterol and fat. Stress is also said to be a cause.

The natural ageing process also contributes to the causation of atherosclerosis.

Signs & Symptoms

If the narrowing of the arteries reduces blood supply to the heart, brain, kidneys, muscles etc., these organs will not function properly, causing angina, hypertension, leg cramps and other disorders.

Further, these narrowings may cause blood to stick to the artery wall and clot there. If the clot is in the heart (thrombosis), it can cause a heart-attack. If it is in the brain circulation, it can cause a stroke.

HOME REMEDIES

1. Garlic is one of the most useful home remedies in this condition. It is useful as a preventive as well as a curative. Many researchers confirmed these benefits.
2. *Rasona Ksheeram* an Ayurvedic formulation, that can be prepared at home is to be taken daily. *Rasona* means garlic and *Ksheeram* indicates milk.

Method of preparation:

Take 5 grams of raw garlic cloves, remove the outer layers and the inside pedicels, and soak in 50ml buttermilk for 6 hours. Then wash and put them in 200 ml of milk. Boil the milk till ¼ of the quantity approximately (i.e., 50ml) is remaining. Filter it and add some sugar if one is not a diabetic and consume as a single dose at bed time daily.

AYURVEDIC REMEDIES

1. *Guglip* is the drug of choice 1 tab. twice daily.
2. *Punarnava Guggulu* 2 tab. twice daily with warm milk or water.

For details on Ayurvedic Standard Medicines, refer to Glossary

5. STROKE

INTRODUCTION

Stroke refers to a clinical condition wherein the blood supply to a part of the brain is suddenly and critically impaired by a blood clot (cerebral thrombosis) or when a ruptured artery leaks blood into the brain (cerebral haemorrhage). The second one is more likely to occur in persons who have high B.P.

In either case, the affected brain cells cease to function.

TREATMENT

Homely Aid for a stroke is merely supportive.

Causative Factors

Each area of the brain controls a different system or part of the body, and the effect of stroke depends on the part/parts of the brain damaged. Major strokes are fatal, but many people make successful recoveries from minor strokes.

Strokes are more common in the persons over 50.

Signs & Symptoms

General
- The symptoms and signs may be confused with DRUNKENNESS.
- There will be sudden and severe headache.

Contd ...

If conscious, lay the person down with head and shoulders slightly raised and supported.

Position head on the side to allow saliva to drain from the mouth.

Rush the person to hospital immediately. During convalescing from a stroke however, home and herbal remedies are highly useful and are applied symptomatically.

- A full, bounding pulse is observed.
- The affected person is disoriented and confused, and may be anxious and weeping.
- Giddiness and possible unconsciousness may occur.

Depending on the extent of the stroke one or more of the following physical defects may occur:

* Paralysis of the mouth — the corner of the mouth may droop, saliva may dribble from it, and speech may be slurred.
* Weakness and decreased sensation in one or both limbs and on one side of the body.
* Flushed face — hot and dry skin.
* Pupils may be unequally dilated.
* Loss of bladder and bowel control.

1. MUSCLE CRAMPS

INTRODUCTION

An involuntary and painful contraction of a voluntary muscle or group of muscles is known as a cramp.

Causative Factors

- Excessive exercise exceeding one's own capacity.
- Indulgence in dry and rough food articles.
- Exposure to cold, taking harmful medicines etc.

TREATMENT

HOME REMEDIES

Massage is the best treatment for relaxation of the contracted muscles. This can be done at home itself. It should be done by rubbing medicated oils on the affected muscles.

Garlic Oil: 10 to 15 Garlic cloves should be crushed and added to 50 ml of any cooking oil and boiled on slow fire till half of the oil remains, and filtered. This is one of the effective home remedies for massage and gives immediate relief.

Those who experience cramps frequently can even use homely gingelly oil and have a massage by themselves, before taking daily bath.

AYURVEDIC REMEDIES

1. Available at Ayurvedic stores for this complaint is *Simhanada Guggul* - 2 tablets which should be taken twice a day with a glass of lukewarm water for 15 days. This will relieve cramps and prevent their recurrence. *Maha Narayana Tailam* is a very effective oil for external application.
2. *Godanti Mishran* - 1 pill three times a day.

_____

For details on Ayurvedic Standard Medicines, refer to Glossary

DO'S & DON'TS

1. Fruits should be taken.
2. Legs should be kept warm in cold seasons.

2. PARKINSON'S DISEASE

INTRODUCTION

Parkinson's disease is that which affects the nervous system. It is also known as Paralysis agitans.

Men are more affected than women. The most vulnerable age group is above 50 years.

PATHOLOGY

Cells called substantia nigra are responsible for producing packets of a chemical called DOPAMINE — a chemical neurotransmitter, that carries signals between the cells. The cells of substantia nigra regularly send dopamine to a second structure in the brain called striatum, which, with the help of dopamine coordinates body movement. Once these cells cease to produce dopamine, the patients' movements too stop.

Luckily, Parkinson's disease can be checked with the help of the drug Leva-dopa, though it does not offer a permanent cure.

TREATMENT

In the early stages, Parkinson's disease is treated with physiotherapy.

AYURVEDIC REMEDIES

Ayurveda recommends a herb known as *Kapi Kachhu*, botanically known as 'Mucuna pruriens', for this disorder. Incidentally, this contains dopamine in natural form, the synthetic version being prescribed in modern medicine. ½ to 1 tsf of the powder well mixed in a cup of milk is given twice a day. There are many useful drugs in Ayurveda for this disease, known as 'Kampa Vata'. The drugs generally used are *Suvarna Bhupati Rasa, Brihat Vata, Chintamani Rasa*. These are gold-based compounds, and are as such to be used under the care of an Ayurvedic physician. The Ayurvedic line of treatment also includes massage with some medicated oils like *Maha Mashadi Tailam* etc. The Ayurvedic approach usually gives good response in many patients, without any ill effects.

Causative Factors

Parkinson's disease is caused by the very gradual deterioration of "junctions", popularly known as ganglia in the nervous system. These junctions are situated at the base of the brain and once affected, affect muscle control and movement in turn. The exact cause for this deterioration is not yet known fully.

Signs & Symptoms

Symptoms usually develop over a long span of time, initially these are unnoticeable.

- Tremors begin in a hand or limb when the muscles are at rest.
- These tremors progressively get worse and spread to both sides of the body.
- As a result, walking may become stiff and unbalanced.
- Posture is usually very stooped and stiff.
- Even simple routine tasks become very difficult and sometimes impossible to perform.
- Depression is common.

Notes * Even though no exact cause is known, there is no evidence that Parkinson's disease is hereditary.
* About 1 person out of 200 has Parkinson's disease.
* Ayurvedic management offers some hope.

3. EPILEPSY

INTRODUCTION

Epilepsy refers to a disorder in which the person has a tendency to have seizures or fits. A seizure is due to abnormal electrical activity of the brain.

TREATMENT

HOME REMEDIES

1. Cow's ghee is used for deep inhalation.
2. Garlic—*Rason Kalp*—a preparation is taken once a day. Garlic strings are crushed and boiled with milk. When reduced to half, it is ready for use.

AYURVEDIC REMEDIES

1. *Brahmivati* is a drug of choice 1-2 pills 2 times a day.
2. Tab. *Mentat* (Himalaya Drugs) 1 tab. three times a day for 6 months to 3 years.
3. *Vacha* powder ½ teaspoonful is also used three times a day.
4. *Brihat-vat-kulantak Ras* is very good in curing epilepsy but should be taken under supervision.
5. *Til* oil or *Brahmi Amla Taila* is good for head massage.

Causative Factors

● Injury to baby during delivery.
● Delay in delivery with decreased oxygen supply to brain.
● Hydrocephalus—excessive fluid in the brain.
● Infections of the brain—meningitis, encephalitis.
● Tumours, tuberculosis, parasites in the brain.
● Drugs e.g. pencillin chloroquine, medicines for depression, angina.

Signs & Symptoms

A typical fit involves movement of one or both limbs of the body with or without loss of consciousness. During the fit some patients lose control of urine and stool. The patient after regaining consciousness, is confused, may have headache and go to sleep.

DO'S & DON'TS

Mental strain of all types should be avoided. Intake of pungent things is strictly prohibited.

4. FACIAL PARALYSIS

INTRODUCTION

The muscles of the face are supplied with nerves which control their actions. These nerves start from the brain and via the skull enter the different parts of the face. Sometimes the facial nerve may be compressed due to inflammation giving rise to paralysis of the facial muscles.

Causative Factors

The cause is not known. It is often caused by exposure to cold wind and improper diet.

Signs & Symptoms

Initially the patient feels the face to be stiff and experiences difficulty in moving it. Taste on the affected side is sometimes affected. The patient cannot close his eyes completely and tears come out. There may be difficulty in eating food and drinking water.

TREATMENT

HOME REMEDIES

1. Garlic is good for paralysis.
2. Cow's ghee and butter milk are also taken daily as much as possible.

AYURVEDIC REMEDIES

1. *Vatagajankusha Ras* 2 pills three times a day in acute cases takes good care. The pill should be crushed and mixed with honey.
2. *Dashmularishta* is very effective on the nervous system. 4 teaspoonfuls of it mixed with equal quantity of water is given twice daily till the symptoms subside.
3. *Maha Narayana Taila* is good for external massage.

For details on Ayurvedic Remedies, refer to Glossary

DO'S & DON'TS

1. The patient should avoid cold things like ice-cream, coca-cola, iced beer and alcoholic liquids.
2. He/she should not be exposed to rain or cold winds.
3. Proper care of eyes should be taken.

5. POOR MEMORY

INTRODUCTION

Memory consists of remembering what has been learnt recently or in the past. Many people have problems in memory which may be a temporary phase (e.g., after a head injury or a fit) or a permanent and progressive disorder.

Causative Factors
Tempory loss of memory is due to:
● Head injury.
● A bout of excessive alcohol.
● A fit.
● Acute anxiety or stress-disorder.
Permanent loss of memory is due to:
● Degenerative diseases e.g., Alzheimer's disease.
● Tumours of the brain.
● Deficiency of vitamin B_1 or B_{12}
● Syphilis, AIDS.
● Chronic alcoholism.

TREATMENT

HOME REMEDIES

1. *Amla* is best for poor memory. Its powder, *murabba*, vegetable can be consumed.
2. 5-10 Almonds should be taken daily.

AYURVEDIC REMEDIES

1. *Brahmi Vati* 1 tab. twice daily with milk after meals.
2. *Tab Mentat* 1 tab. three times a day.
3. *Brahmighrita* one teaspoonful twice daily with milk.
4. Tab. *Brento* (Ban) 1 tab. twice daily.

_____

For details on Ayurvedic Standard Medicines, refer to Glossary

DO'S & DON'TS

1. The patient should be kept free from worries, anxieties, emotional stress.
2. Meditation proves useful in correcting and promoting memory.

6. HYSTERIA

INTRODUCTION

Hysteria is usually caused by a reaction to an emotional upset or nervous stress and is likely to be aggravated by onlookers.

TREATMENT

1. Isolate the affected person from any onlookers and gently but firmly help to calm him/her enough to regain control.
2. Reassure the patient, but refrain from showing any sympathy and, gently but firmly, escort him/her to a quiet place.
   Do not physically restrain or slap the person, this may make the patient turn more aggressive/violent.
3. Stay with patient and keep under observation until full recovery takes place.
4. Arrange for medical aid.

HOME REMEDIES

Asafoetida: Popularly known as *hing*, for medical use, asafoetida should be roasted with a little pure ghee on a hot pan. This process removes impurities. Regular use of asafoetida strengthens the nervous system. 1gm of purified *hing* should be given with luke warm water to hysteria affected persons for 40 days.

Pure Ghee: It is of great value in the treatment of hysteria. It can be given with rice or chapatis. 5gms of pure cow ghee well mixed in a glass of warm milk can be given, preferably at bed-time.

Almonds: Almonds are very useful for hysterical patients. Two almonds soaked in water overnight, should be made into a paste, with a little sugar and taken regularly once a day to improve the mental make-up of the affected person.

AYURVEDIC REMEDIES

1. *Brahmivati* available in tablet form, should be taken in the dose of 1 tablet twice a day with water.
2. *Ashwagandha Churna* is another simple herbal remedy. 5gms of powder well mixed in 10gms of pure ghee should be taken along with a cup of warm milk at bedtime.
3. *Mentat* tablet (Himalaya Drugs) 1 tablet twice daily with water given for 2 to 3 months strengthens the nervous system.
4. *Brento* tablet (Ban) is also very useful in the dosage as above.

DO'S & DON'TS

Dhyana and *Yoga* are essential to build-up the inner self control as only the weak minded are susceptible to this disorder.

Causative Factors

It is the consequential effect of suppressed conflicts within the person. It is more common in young women in the age group of 15-30 years.

Signs & Symptoms

- Temporary loss of behavioural control is seen in the individual with dramatic shouting, screaming, crying and wild beating of limbs. The affected may roll on the ground and tear hair and clothes.
- Hysterical over-breathing (hyperventilation) may follow.
- The affected may be unable to move or be walking strangely for no apparent reason.

7. SCHIZOPHRENIA

INTRODUCTION

Schizophrenia is a major psychiatric (mental) illness which is chronic in nature and affects the social and personal life of the patient.

TREATMENT

HOME REMEDIES

Saffron is very useful for it. Two-four strings of it are to be boiled with milk and given to patient early in the morning.

AYURVEDIC REMEDIES

1. The powder of *Jatamansi* one tsf three times a day.
2. *Vatakulantak Ras* ½ tab. three times a day.
3. *Vacha, Shankhpushpi, Sarpagandha* are also used together or separately.
4. *Dhara* with medicated oil also proves useful.

Causative Factors

It is normally due to abnormal secretion of two chemical substances in the brain i.e., serotonin and dopamine. It is known to run in families. Stress is a precipitating factor. It is seen in the age-group of 15 to 25 years.

Signs & Symptoms

Signs and symptoms vary according to the type of schizophrenia. The common symptoms are suspiciousness, lack of socialization, not taking care of self, not going to work, abnormal behaviour, hallucinations (seeing, hearing, or smelling things) and false beliefs.

DO'S & DON'TS

Since it is a psychic disease, it is best treated with psycho-therapy.

8. INSOMNIA/SLEEPING PROBLEMS

INTRODUCTION

Insomnia means difficulty in getting sleep, disturbed sleep or waking in the early hours of the morning and being unable to get back to sleep.

HOME REMEDIES

Green *dhaniya* (Coriandrum sativum) in the form of 15ml of its expressed juice, well mixed with sugar and water induces sleep. Since lack of physical activity seems to be one of the causes, regular exercise helps relieve sleeplessness to a great extent.

AYURVEDIC REMEDIES

1. Before going to bed, have a head massage with a herbal medicated oil, *Brahmi tailam* and have a cup full of warm milk with some *Brahmivati*, a herbal malted milk drink.
2. *Aswagandha Churna,* a readymade drug in powder form is very useful in this condition. 5 grams of the powder should be taken with sugar and ghee twice a day after meals.
3. Drinking *amla* juice 15-20ml before going to bed is also useful.
4. *Brahmivati* 2 tablets at bedtime taken with a cup of warm milk induces good sleep.
5. *Sunidra* tablet (Maharishi Ayurved) 1 to 2 tablets at bedtime acts as a tranquilizer.
6. *Calmtone* capsule (Uttam) 1 to 2 capsules twice daily after meals is very useful in this condition.
7. *Shirodhara*—a part of *Panchkarma* is also very useful in chronic insomnia.

| Causative Factors |

Domestic worries are the usual cause. Over-excitement, ill-health, or depression may also be the causes.

Sometimes withdrawal of sleeping tablets also leads to this problem. Even if one consumes stimulants such as caffeine late in the evening, he may be susceptible to this problem.

| Signs & Symptoms |

Not having enough sleep constantly. Not every body, however requires the same amount of sleep. On an average 8 hours sleep is ideal, but some persons need more and others far less.

9. HEADACHE

INTRODUCTION

Headache is probably the most common complaint, yet it is difficult to define or treat accurately, that is why in the medical world very often it is repeated that treatment of headache is quite a headache for the doctor. Even though a good majority of headaches are quite harmless, a few ones may indicate a grave disorder like a brain tumour. As such one should consult a competent doctor, in case the headache is continuous and not responding to common remedies.

TREATMENT

HOME REMEDIES

Heena: The tender flowers of *Henna* should be rubbed to a pasty consistency and applied over the forehead for relief.

Jalebi: An easily available sweet, it is of great help in headache. Immerse 2 to 3 *Jalebis* in a glass of warm milk for a few minutes, then drink the mixture once or twice a day.

Cinnamon: It can be used for external application. A fine paste of this spice should be made by adding few drops of water on a stone. This has to be applied over the temples and forehead to obtain relief.

AYURVEDIC REMEDIES

1. *Sootasekhara Rasa* 1 tablet along with 3gm of *Sitopaladi Churna,* should be taken twice a day with a cup of warm milk. This resolves all routine headaches.
2. *Godanti Mishran,* a readymade compound drug available in tablet form, can be taken orally twice a day with some lukewarm water.
3. *Pathyadi Quatham,* an oral liquid, 15ml twice a day with equal water is also a good remedy.
4. Many pain balms available in the market are Ayurvedic drugs. As such they can also be tried for external applications.
5. *Shirshuladi Vajra Ras* is very useful in general headache.
6. Cephagraine tablet (Charak) 1 tablet thrice daily for 2 weeks along with cephagraine nasal drops 2 to 4 drops before sunrise give immediate relief even in cases of migraine.

For details on Ayurvedic Standard Medicines, refer to Glossary

OTHER MEASURES

DIET: Affected persons should avoid cold items like curd, ice creams, cold water, cold drinks and should not take bath in cold water, or get exposed to cold climatic conditions as this may aggravate the headache.

Causative Factors

The causes are so varied that it is often difficult to locate the exact cause, or the physical or emotional problem at the root of the trouble, such as various kinds of tension, fatigue, anxiety or emotional upsets.

In some instances, the headache may reflect some disorder of infection settled somewhere in the body, or accompany a problem affecting the eyes, sinuses, teeth or neck.

Signs & Symptoms

The headache experienced can vary in intensity from mild discomfort to very severe, stabbing pain.

10. FATIGUE

(General debility)

INTRODUCTION

Because of excessive and prolonged durations of work, everyone experiences a feeling of complete exhaustion occasionally, which is known as fatigue.

HOME REMEDIES

Fruits: Fruit juices are generally helpful in this condition.

1. Grape juice is specially useful as it immediately brings in stamina.
2. Dates or *Khajura* are great sources of instant energy. These should be taken regularly along with a glass of milk.
3. Nutritious food should be taken and fried and junk foods avoided.

Exercise: Improvement of blood circulation is necessary to combat fatigue. This can be achieved by daily exercise routines like brisk walks, gardening, taking up a sport, or swimming.

AYURVEDIC REMEDIES

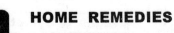

1. *Ashwagandha Churna* — 5gms twice a day, well mixed in a glass of milk should be taken regularly. It is a good health supplement.
2. *Geriforte* tablet (Himalaya Drugs) 1 tab. twice daily. Not to be used in people with high blood pressure.
3. *Trasina* capsule (Dey's) 1 capsule twice daily for 7 days.
4. *Aswal Plus* capsule 1 capsule twice daily.

For details on Ayurvedic Standard Medicines, refer to Glossary

1. ACNE AND PIMPLES

INTRODUCTION

Acne is a very common problem affecting teenagers. It is a skin complaint in which spots, blackheads and pimples appear on the face, neck and body.

HEALING HINTS

1. Wash frequently with soap and water.
2. Do not prick or squeeze the pimples with bare fingers.
3. Use a special blackhead-extractor.
4. Avoid excessive fatty & oily food stuff.
5. Sandalwood, turmeric, aloe, and *neem* are the best home remedies.

TREATMENT

HOME REMEDIES

1. The paste made of *Jeera* (cumin seeds) applied over the pimples gives relief. For a single application, 5gm of *Jeera* is sufficient to prepare the paste. After one hour, the application can be removed.
2. The paste of 5gm each of red sandalwood (*Rakta Chandan*) and turmeric made with milk is a very efficacious local application.
3. Cumin seeds popularly known as *ajwain* are also useful in this condition. Prepare the paste of 5gm *ajwain*, duly adding required quantity of water and apply on the face.
4. *Kumari* pulp (known as Aloe vera) should be taken internally. Extracted juice of Aloe vera (half a cup) should be taken internally twice a day.

Causative Factors

At the root of the problem are the sebaceous glands, which secrete an oily fluid known as sebum. During teenage, the hormonal changes taking place stimulate these glands to produce larger quantities of sebum than before, thus making the skin greasier.

The problem erupts if the exit to the gland (in the hair follicle) becomes blocked. The sebum begins to "back-up" in the gland, causing it to swell slightly, and this plug at exit may turn black on contact with air, so causing a blackhead. This is not due to dirt but is due to a chemical process known as Oxidation. If bacteria and sebum are trapped inside the gland by the plug, the tissues become inflamed and form a pimple.

5. Fresh juice of tender *tulsi* leaves (Ocimum basilicum) is to be applied externally daily.
6. The paste of *jatiphal* (nutmeg) made with water is also very useful.

AYURVEDIC REMEDIES

1. *Kumkumadi Lepam,* an ointment for application over the face, after duly washing the face can be used daily until pimples disappear.
2. Some herbal blood purifying drugs may also be taken for better results. *Saribadyasava* 15 to 30ml taken after meals with equal quantity of water, twice a day helps in the cure of acne vulgaris.
3. RS Forte syrup (DAP) is a good oral liquid for this condition. 20ml of syrup well mixed with 20ml of cold water should be taken orally twice a day for 40 days for good results.
4. Skinelle tablets (Charak Pharma) taken orally along with Skinelle ointment applied externally produce very good results in just two weeks.
5. Acnenil capsules (Uttam Pharma) in the dose of one capsule thrice daily after meals for a fortnight is a useful remedy for acne.
6. *Jeevan Amrit (Neem* oil) capsules taken once daily on an empty stomach help in curing acne and blackheads.
7. Rasana Forte capsules (Shilpa Chem), an extract of garlic should be taken orally twice daily for 20 to 30 days.
8. *Trifala Churna* taken 5 to 10 gm daily helps in purifying the blood thus helping in the cure of acne.
9. Clean-N-Clear syrup (Dabur) should be taken 1 teaspoonful thrice daily after meals for a month.

For details on Ayurvedic Standard Medicines, refer to Glossary

DO'S & DON'TS

1. Constipation, if present should be tackled effectively. For this 5gm/1 tsp of *Swadista Virechana Churna* should be taken at bed time along with a glass of water. This ensures safe bowel movement.
2. Associated dandruff should be treated.

2. DANDRUFF

INTRODUCTION

Dandruff is a harmless disease of the skin/scalp, wherein a thin mica like scaling, which aggravates on scratching, occurs along with acute burning and itching sensation. Papules are rough and itching having no discharge. Though this condition may occur at any age, it is very common among the young.

DO'S & DON'TS

1. Dandruff is the most common cause of hair fall.
2. Hygiene and cleanliness of combs is essential as reinfection is common.
3. Do not wash hair too often.

TREATMENT

HOME REMEDIES

1. Clean the hair 2 or 3 times a week with a mildly medicated shampoo.
2. The emulsion prepared with the oil of sandalwood and lemon juice is highly effective. One part of sandalwood oil is mixed with three parts of fresh lemon juice and briskly shaken in a glass bottle before applying.
3. Application of a mixture of *neem* oil and camphor is also effective, followed by washing the hair.
4. Some internal medicines for blood purification and relieving itching sensation may be used as and when required.
5. About 25gm of dry *amla* is soaked in a litre of water overnight. It is boiled in the morning until half of it remains. To this 25gm of yoghurt is added and the paste applied on the scalp. After one hour the paste is washed first with *amla* water and then plain water. This procedure should be repeated every week for 2 to 3 months.
6. Decoction of bark of a *neem* tree is also useful for external application.
7. Coconut oil mixed with lemon juice is very effective for external usage.

Causative Factors

The actual cause of dandruff is not clear, but some doctors believe it is the result of either too much or too little oil being produced by sebaceous glands in the scalp.

Sometimes there is an underlying fungal infection of the scalp. Dandruff appears when the skin on the scalp sheds its dead cells rather more quickly and profusely than usual. It is usually worst on greasy skins.

Signs & Symptoms

Dry white scales are shed on the clothes. Occasionally, dandruff can develop into a more severe seborrhoeic dermatitis, the signs of which are a reddened, greasy and very itchy scalp with brownish scales in the hair.

AYURVEDIC REMEDIES

Popular Ayurvedic safe drugs indicated for dandruff are:

1. *Brihat Haridra Khanda* available in powder form can be taken in a dose of 1½ teaspoonful well mixed in a glass of milk twice a day. This powder not only cures the dandruff but also improves the complexion and colour.

2. Blood purifying oral liquids are *Khadirarista* and *Saribadyasavam*. Any one of them or both together can be taken internally twice a day preferably after meals. Dose is 20ml medicine well mixed in 20ml of water.

3. *Bhringaraj Tailam* applied externally and *Bhringaraj Churna* (½ teaspoonful twice daily) taken internally cure dandruff within a month.

4. Septilin tablets (Himalaya Drugs) in the dose of one tablet twice daily can be taken if there is any infection of the scalp. This medicine should not be used by pregnant women.

5. Purified powder of sulphur *(Gandhak Rasayana)* 60mg twice daily mixed with honey or butter can be taken by mouth for fungal infection and dandruff of long duration.

For details on Ayurvedic Standard Medicines, refer to Glossary

3. HAIR FALL AND GREYING OF HAIR

INTRODUCTION

Hair fall and greying of hair at an early stage of life can be very embarassing, especially for young girls and boys who develop a feeling of social stigma.

TREATMENT

HOME REMEDIES

1. First and foremost, the scalp of the affected person should be energetically massaged daily for 10 to 15 minutes with fingers, after cleaning it with water. This mechanical action activates the hair follicles by ensuring blood circulation, and warms up the scalp.

Causative Factors

Inadequate nutrition is the main causative factor for hairfall and greying of hair in the lower classes. Sometimes even a partial lack of B-vitamins and folic acid leads to hair fall and baldness. In such cases hair regrows after treatment with vitamins.

Stress, worry, and anxiety are the important psychological factors, especially in youngsters for these disorders.

Chronic diseases like anaemia, cold, flu, syphilis, tuberculosis, and

Contd ...

2. *Amla* Hair Oil: *Amla* hair oil can be made at home itself, by adding fresh juice of Indian gooseberries to pure coconut oil. This should be boiled till the *Amla* juice is completely absorbed in the oil. This oil should be applied after the above said massage.

3. The powder of *amla* and *Bhringaraj* is also used internally in a dose of one teaspoonful thrice daily with milk or water.

4. The pulp of *amla* and mango mixed together is used externally on the scalp.

radiation therapy also account for hair loss and baldness.

Conditions like psoriasis, dandruff and other fungal infections also cause hair loss considerably.

Sometimes a heriditary factor runs in the family members, which remains unresponsive to any kind of treatment.

AYURVEDIC REMEDIES

1. Some medicated hair oil available over the counter for hair fall are:
   a. *Neeli Bhringamalaka Tailam*   Any one of these oils should be applied
   b. *Bhringáraj Tailam*   onto the scalp, twice a week at bedtime.
   c. *Brahmi Amla Kesha Tailam*

Regular washing of the hair with *shikakai* is a must and soap should be avoided. Greying of hair and hair fall stops in many cases, after 2 to 3 months usage of these oils.

2. Combination of *Bhringaraj Churna* ½ teaspoonful thrice daily and *Bhringaraj* capsule, one capsule twice daily with water after meals along with *Bhringaraj Tailam* locally yields very good results.

3. *Shad Bindu Tailam* is used for inhalation (Nasya) once daily for 1 to 2 months.

4. *Neem* oil is also used for inhalation twice daily for about a month. Along with this only milk is taken in the diet.

5. *Triphala Churna* taken 5 to 10gm at bedtime with milk or water for a long time can prove very effective in curing greying and falling of hair.

6. Hair sure oil (Platinum Remedies) is also very good.

7. Sesa oil (Ban) proves very useful if used for 3 months.

For details on Ayurvedic Standard Medicines, refer to Glossary

DO'S & DON'TS

For Baldness

After regular rubbing of the scalp as stated earlier a special oil HAIR RICH OIL should be applied on the scalp and rubbed further, till scalp becomes warm. This promotes hair to regrow, though slowly.

Proper diet, peace of mind, and healthy lifestyle components as detailed in the chapter 'TIPS FOR POSITIVE HEALTH' are essential in these conditions of premature greying, hair fall, and baldness.

4. BOILS

INTRODUCTION

Boils are painful, red, pus-filled swellings that are formed in any part of the body. These are caused by a type of bacterium that lives silently on the surface of the skin.

People who suffer from eczema or any problem that affects the structure of the skin's surface are more prone or susceptible to boils or carbuncles.

Carbuncles are simply large boils or a collection of boils joined together.

TREATMENT

HOME REMEDIES

1. Dry ginger and asafoetida (i.e., *sonth* and *hing*) paste should be made by adding a small quantity of water. This paste should be applied over the areas of boils twice a day as an external measure.
2. Turmeric powder paste should be made by adding *tulsi* leaves' juice. This should be applied over the boils.
3. The same combination can also be taken internally. These are proven anti-bacterials as well as good blood purifiers.
4. Betel leaves: A leaf is gently warmed till it becomes soft and then coated with a layer of pure castor oil. This processed betel leaf should be spread over the inflamed part. This should be repeated thrice a day. After a few applications, the boil will rupture.
5. The root of *Shobanjan (Sehjana)* and *Devdaru* crushed is mixed with *kanji* and made in the form of a paste. This when applied over the inflamed part gives immediate results. This is also called *Shobanjanadi Lepam*.
6. A paste of mustard seeds also produces results at its earliest.

Causative Factors

- Boils are basically caused by bacteria, (staphylococcus) which enter the sweat glands or hair follicles.
- They are sometimes caused by blood impurities.
- The boil first appears when the bacteria start to multiply under the skin and produce toxic chemicals, which inflame the surrounding area.
- In an effort to combat these chemicals, more and more white blood cells rush to the spot of infection until a pocket of pus is formed in the skin.
- This pocket becomes the centre of the boil.

Signs & Symptoms

Boils usually develop on the legs, arms and trunk. The first symptom is a small, red, painful area of skin, which may be slightly swollen.

As the pus starts to form, the centre becomes yellow and the pain and swelling increase.

AYURVEDIC REMEDIES

1. *Kanchanara Guggulu* is the suitable remedy, in doses of 2 pills twice a day.
2. *Maha Manjista Quatham* an oral liquid, 20ml of which when given with equal quantity of water twice a day, provides great relief.
3. *Triphalachurna*: 10gms of this powder should be added to 50ml of hot water and kept for some time. This should be taken at bedtime. This relieves constipation, and makes bowel movements free.
4. *Nityanand Ras* 250mg mixed with a bit of honey can be given thrice a day.
5. *Kaishora Guggulu* in the dose of 1 to 2 pills 2 to 3 times daily is useful.
6. *Shatavari Ghritam* 5 to 10ml with milk given twice daily is a good remedy for boils.
7. Skinelle tablets (Charak) 1 to 2 tablets twice or thrice daily for 7 to 10 days can cure the boils.
8. *Charmardadi Tailam* is useful for external use.

5. BURNS

INTRODUCTION

Burns cause serious injury to body tissues caused by heat, chemicals or radiation. However heat is the most common cause. There is severe risk of infection with burns because it damages the skin's protection against germs.

> ### Signs & Symptoms
> A minor burn causes painful reddening and blistering. A severe burn leaves a painless white or charred area.

Even though there are a number of classifications of burns, area and depth-wise classification is important from treatment point of view.

Area: The area of burn gives a rough guide as to whether or not a casualty is likely to suffer shock. The greater the area involved, the higher the possibility of shock, because of greater fluid loss. For example an average adult with a superficial burn covering 9% or more of the body surface will need hospitalisation.

TREATMENT

The affected area should be placed immediately under a steady flow of cold water for at least 10 minutes or until the pain stops. If a blister forms, it should not be pricked as it will leave the raw skin open for infection.

HOME REMEDIES

1. Spread a thin layer of the pulp of Aloe vera, (a jelly like substance) or its juice over the affected area twice a day.
2. Pure turmeric powder can also be applied with some honey.
3. The ointment prepared from the ash of dry coconut and coconut oil is a very useful application over burns.

AYURVEDIC REMEDIES

1. *Sindooradi Lepa,* a market preparation available in the ointment form can also be applied over the burnt areas to prevent infections.
2. The mixture of the white of an egg and the powder of the gum of the *babul* tree with coconut oil is applied as an ointment over the burn.
3. The juice extracted from the stem of plantain tree can also be applied.
4. In case of severe and major burns, medical attention is required. Only minor burns should be treated with home remedies.

BURNING SENSATION

It is usually felt on the palms and soles.

HOME REMEDIES

1. The poultice of henna *(mehndi)* leaves made with vinegar *(kanjee)* or lemon juice is very useful and gives prompt relief.
2. The paste made of the leaves of Vitex nigundo *(Nirgundi)* applied on the feet gives quick relief.
3. The ointment prepared with pure ghee 250gm mixed with 12gm each of *raal* and white *jeera* gives immediate relief.

For details, refer to Part III, Glossary.

AYURVEDIC REMEDIES

1. *Hima Sagara Taila* is a specific medicated oil to be applied over burning feet. It immediately cures the burning sensation and is easily available at Ayurvedic stores.
2. *Chandanadi Taila* is also useful for application.

6. CORN

INTRODUCTION

Corns and calluses are areas of skin that have been thickened because of constant pressure. The difference between corns and calluses is that corns are small and arise on the toes, while calluses are bigger and generally develop on the soles of the feet.

STRUCTURE

A corn looks like a hardened yellowish mass, and may or may not be painful, but there is always a danger that it may become a problem at a later stage.

Causative Factors

Everybody at some or other point of time may face these problems. These develop as a sequel to wearing ili-fitting or worn-out shoes or hard & firm slippers. These cause patches of thickened, hardened skin at the various points where shoes exert friction or pressure on the skin surface.

TREATMENT

HOME REMEDIES

1. Since these are hardened masses, a gentle application of castor oil or coconut oil on these spots regularly 3 to 4 times a day makes them soft.
2. Turmeric powder well mixed in honey or *neem* oil should be applied on these corns.
3. Temporary use of an insole or a replaceable pad to wear inside a shoe—to relieve excess pressure on the foot is essential.
4. The milky juice of papaya fruit is applied to remove corns.

AYURVEDIC REMEDIES

Kasisadi Taila is a readymade preparation. It is to be applied on the corns for a few days until the corns become soft and ultimately fall out.

7. ECZEMA

INTRODUCTION

There are numerous skin diseases, which are inadequately treated by modern medicine, and eczema is one such problem. Eczema means a 'boiling over' of the skin and is characterised by spontaneous eruptions with mild to severe itching, redness, flaking and tiny blisters.

In chronic cases, the skin becomes thickened and appears like the 'bark of a tree'.

TREATMENT

The causative factors should be avoided.

HOME REMEDIES

1. The affected part should be cleaned daily with warm water boiled with the bark of the *neem* tree. This simple measure prevents secondary infections, and itching.
2. The paste prepared from *neem* bark should be applied on the affected part and allowed to dry and then washed off.
3. Pure *neem* oil, in a dosage of 2 to 4 drops well mixed in a cup of warm milk with sugar should be taken daily for 40 days.
4. *Doob* grass, *harar*, *sendha namak*, *chakbar* and *tulsi* taken in equal quantities and crushed with *kanji* or buttermilk and applied on affected areas daily for 4 to 6 weeks gives good results.

AYURVEDIC REMEDIES

A number of effective, soothing ointment/oils are available which are to be used under the supervision of an Ayurvedic physician, since these contain arsenic, mercury, suphur, etc.

Causative Factors

- Allergic reaction
- Inherited Stress or
- A combination of the above

Signs & Symptoms

- Infant eczema: A child may show signs of eczema at a very tender age of a few months after birth. A rash appears on the face, and may spread to the rest of the body, and the child suffers severe itching.
- Contact eczema: After contact with a substance to which one is allergic—for example, jewellery, certain plants or cosmetics, a person gets this type of eczema. The skin becomes red and itchy with tiny blisters starting to appear within 48 hours of contact.
- Housewife's eczema: It is an irritant eczema caused by prolonged exposure of the hands to detergents, washing liquids, shampoos and other cosmetic items. In this variety the skin may crack, flake and itch.

Some simple safe and pure herbal preparations of Ayurveda are listed below.

1. *Pancha Tikta Ghrita Guggul* — A *ghee* based pure herbal preparation — 2 teaspoonfuls well mixed in a cup of hot milk, should be taken on empty stomach, preferably in the early morning, followed by some warm water.
2. *Khadirarishta,* an oral liquid in doses of 20ml well mixed with equal quantity of water — should be taken twice a day after meals.
3. For external application, *Guduchyadi Tailam*, a medicated oil can be applied on the patches as a primary drug.
4. Skinille tablets (Charak) 1 to 2 tablets 2 to 3 times a day with water after meals are very useful for treating eczema.
5. Raktoplen tablets (Bharat Ayurvedic Pharmacy) 1 to 2 tablets twice or thrice daily act as a blood purifier and control infection.
6. *Mahamarichayadi Tailam* is very effective for external application.
7. *Panchnimbadi Churna* ½ to 1 teaspoon twice daily taken with water after meals gives very good results in 15 to 20 days.
8. Safi, a popular blood-purifier is taken 1 to 2 teaspoons on an empty stomach and helps in curing eczema.

For details on Ayurvedic Standard Medicines, refer to Glossary

DO'S & DON'TS

1. Avoid contact with detergent; if unavoidable, wear cotton gloves & wash.
2. Keep the eczema patches free from any tight clothing.
3. Avoid use of synthetic clothing which prevent evaporation of sweat.
4. Eat water melon fruit daily.
5. Aviod sour things like pickles, curds, meat, fish and eggs.
6. Pure turmeric & neem are the choice home remedies.

DIETS

1. Sour items like pickles and curds are to be avoided.
2. Bitter gourd and *neem* flowers are highly beneficial.
3. Pure turmeric is extremely useful; it can be applied externally over the patches and can be taken internally along with milk in a dose of ½ teaspoonful twice a day.

8. URTICARIA

INTRODUCTION

Urticaria is a common reaction pattern characterized by the presence of swelling of different parts of body and lasting for less than 24 hours.

Causative Factors

- Allergens in food.
- Heat/cold pressure, exercise.
- Jaundice.
- Pregnancy.
- Intestinal worms.
- Medicines—painkillers, antibiotics, antihypertensives, codeine.

Signs & Symptoms

Urticaria is associated with diffuse swelling of the tongue or throat. It may occur anywhere on the body. Sometimes breathlessness, abdominal pain, headache and even life-threatening shock can occur.

TREATMENT

HOME REMEDIES

1. *Haridra* is a popular home remedy. The powder should be taken ½ tsf twice daily with water.
2. *Gairika* (red ochre) is another popularly used remedy in this condition. One tsf of it mixed with honey taken three times a day.

AYURVEDIC REMEDIES

1. *Sutsekhara Rasa* (simple) 1 tab. three times a day.
2. *Kamdudha Ras* 1 tab. (of 125 mg) 1 tab three times a day.
3. *Haridra Khand* 1 teaspoonful mixed with warm cup of milk at bedtime.
4. Urtiplex tablet (Charak) 1 tab. 4-6 times a day.

DO'S & DON'TS

1. In acute cases mustard oil mixed with salt should be applied over the body.
2. The patient should be dewormed.

9. LEUCODERMA

INTRODUCTION

Vitiligo, also known as leucoderma, is an embarrassing skin disease, wherein white patches occur all over the body including face, scalp and private parts. This causes a lot of mental agony in the affected persons, especially in the youngsters. There is gradual loss of skin pigment called melanin from the layers of the skin.

TREATMENT

HOME REMEDIES

1. A paste made out of *Bakuchi* (Psoralea corylifolia) and vinegar should be applied over the white patches and exposed to early sun-rays for 15 minutes.
2. Ginger juice 10ml twice a day ensures proper blood supply to these white patches.
3. Red clay being rich in copper is effective in the patches. This should be well mixed in fresh ginger juice in equal proportion and applied over the lesions once daily.
4. Turmeric powder well mixed in mustard oil is also a good external application in this disorder.
5. The leaves of *neem* crushed with *amla churna* taken ½ to 1 teaspoonful once daily for about a month shows good results.
6. The decoction of *amla* and *kher* mixed with a small quantity of honey taken in the dose of 20 to 50ml once or twice daily proves very effective.

Causative Factors

- It is not caused by any germs or infective agents.
- The exact causative factor is not known.
- Excessive thinking, worry, chronic gastric problems, improper liver functions, worms/parasites in the digestive system, aggravate 'Vitiligo'.
- Burns and injuries are the other causative factors.
- Heredity is also one of the factors.

Signs & Symptoms

- Initially small white spots appear, and gradually develop into white patches. These can occur all over the body.
- These patches are pale in the beginning, later on they become whiter with time, as the 'melanin' pigment is worn-out from the skin.

AYURVEDIC REMEDIES

1. *Aarogyavardhini* 125mg (pill) should be given twice a day after meals.
2. *Khadirarishta* an oral liquid in a dose of 15ml with 15ml water is given along with *Aarogyavardhini*.
3. *Shwet Kushtahar* capsule orally 1 to 2 capsules twice daily along with *shwet kushtahar vati* for local application cures leucoderma if taken for 4 to 6 months.

For details on Ayurvedic Standard Medicines, refer to Glossary

10. PSORIASIS

INTRODUCTION

Psoriasis is a chronic and recurring skin disorder. It usually occurs between the ages of 14 and 24 and persists for life. However if proper Ayurvedic treatment is initiated in the early stages itself one can restrict the severity and frequency of attacks.

COMPONENTS OF PSORIASIS

1. Hereditary
2. Extreme stress
3. Triggering factors like viral infections/ immunisation.

DO'S & DON'TS

1. Blood purification with drugs/diets.
2. Emotional calm with *Yoga & Dhyana* (prayer).
3. Avoid hot spicy things, curd.
4. Take rocksalt instead of common salt.
5. Bitter things are better things.

TREATMENT

HOME REMEDIES

1. Make fine powder of dried *neem* leaves and store in a clean bottle. Take 1 teaspoonful (5gm) with a glass of water twice a day. This preparation is also available as *Neem* capsule in the Ayurvedic store.
2. Half a teaspoonful of pure *Haldi* powder (i.e., turmeric) is added to the 1 teaspoon ful of *neem* powder, and taken twice a day with lukewarm water.
3. External application of *Karanja Tailam* (Pongamia pinnata) is very effective.

Causative Factors

The exact cause still remains a mystery, some cases may be triggered by viral infections, immunisation or a period of extreme stress.

Psoriasis has a hereditary component, some people can be carriers, i.e., they pass on the disease, even if they do not actually show the symptoms themselves.

In women, the condition may clear up in pregnancy but unfortunately it often reappears after the birth of the baby.

Signs & Symptoms

Although the condition may occur on any part of the body, the characteristic sites are knees and elbows.

There are several different types of psoriatic rashes, the most common one being deep red or purple. The skin is thick and is covered with a silvery scale, which is a diagnostic index.

It can affect any part of the body although it rarely attacks the face.

In Ayurvedic system of medicine, it is known as *Kitibha*. Blood impurities associated with some emotional factors are listed as the causative factors for psoriasis.

Since there is severe irritation of the patches the patient is unable to resist scratching. On scratching scales sometimes watery exudation and blood come out of the patches, which produce a burning sensation.

4. Make a paste of tender neem leaves and little bit of pure turmeric powder. This should be applied over the affected areas before taking bath. The person afflicted with psoriasis should take bath with water boiled in *neem* leaves after the above stated application.

AYURVEDIC REMEDIES

1. *Pancha Tikta Ghrita Guggul* 5gm to 10gm with oral liquid drug of *Maha Manjisthadi*. *Quath* (30ml) should be taken every morning and evening for 40 days.
2. *Maha Tikta Ghritam* also can be taken on the similar lines, if there is no response to the above stated remedy.
3. Oil 777 is meant for application over the patches. After application the affected parts should be exposed to the early morning sunlight for 10 minutes daily.
4. Raktoplex tablet (Bharat Ayurvedic Pharmacy) in the dose of 1 to 2 tablets twice or thrice daily is very useful for psoriasis.
5. *Vikosarsa* tablet 1 to 2 tablets 2 to 3 times daily with water or milk after meals is a good treatment for psoriasis.

For details on Ayurvedic Standard Medicines, refer to Glossary

11. SCABIES

INTRODUCTION

Scabies is one of the most common skin diseases and affects people of either sex at any age.

Generally more than one members of a family are involved due to its infectious nature.

PREVENTION

Scabies and other skin problems can be safely prevented by daily application of a simple Ayurvedic paste which can be made at home.

Signs & Symptoms
The chief complaint is itching which is severe at night. The most common sites or areas affected are:
● The webs of the fingers and toes
● External genitals
● Buttocks
● Front of the wrists and
● Back of the elbows

Paste of *neem* leaves and turmeric in green gram flour and mustard oil in proportions of 1 part *neem*, 1 part turmeric, 8 parts gram flour and oil should be mixed as much as necessary to make it into a paste form.

HOME REMEDIES

1. All clothes of the affected person should be washed in hot water daily. Nails should be trimmed.
2. The areas of the body affected with scabies should be washed with hot water boiled with *neem* leaves and *neem* soap should be used.
3. Tender *neem* leaves, which are not very bitter are made into paste of the size of a 500mg pill and given twice a day.

AYURVEDIC REMEDIES

1. *Maha Marichadi Taila*: A readymade medicated oil available at Ayurvedic stores is the drug of choice in scabies.
   After a good bath with *neem* soap, this oil should be well applied on all parts of the body. This should be continued at least for a week.
2. *Brahmivati* pills are effective in scabies in doses of a 125mg pill twice a day with water.
3. Purified sulphur *(Gandhak)* is commonly used in the treatment of scabies.

METHOD OF PURIFYING SULPHUR

Take 2gm of raw sulphur in a big spoon and to this pure *ghee* (preferably from cow's milk) is added so that the sulphur powder gets fully submerged in it. Put the spoon on fire and heat it. When the *ghee* starts boiling, the sulphur starts melting and is mixed with the *ghee*. Take cow's milk in another pot and cover it with a thin cloth. The hot *ghee* containing sulphur is poured on the cloth. The sulphur comes down in the milk and gets solidified. It is taken out of milk and washed with warm water. This process is repeated seven times. By this process the sulphur becomes pure and is ready for use.

This is given 60-120mg twice daily mixed with honey.

12. SUN BURN

INTRODUCTION

Direct exposure to the sun's rays may produce:
1. Redness,
2. Itching, and
3. Tenderness of the skin.

Signs & Symptoms
• Skin becomes red, tender and swollen with possible blistering.
• Affected skin will feel hot.

It may cause superficial burning to a more severe reaction in which the skin becomes red, blistered and painful.

TREATMENT

1. Remove the person to a cool place and arrange medical aid, if burns are severe.
2. Cool the skin by sponging gently with cold water.

HOME REMEDIES

1. Give the person sips of cold water at frequent intervals.
2. Apply the paste prepared from *chandan* (sandalwood) and *haldi* (turmeric) lightly over the area and replace the application twice a day with freshly prepared paste.
3. 1 teaspoonful of this *(chandan+haldi)* mixture should also be given internally twice a day.
4. Do not break blisters.

13. WARTS

INTRODUCTION

These are harmless growths on the skin or mucous membrane. They can grow upto 6mm in diameter. These appear rough, with a cauliflower-like surface and may have small, black splinter like dots.

Causative Factors

All warts are caused by a virus. This virus is contagious and is spread by touch or through contact.

Signs & Symptoms

The first sign of a wart is usually a small, horny lump on the head, face, scalp or knees, although they can grow on any part of the body.

HOME REMEDIES

Castor oil, if applied regularly for a fairly long period, softens the warts. This should be applied adequately.

Papaya Milk: Papaya fruit milk is also effective in breaking the warts. Its regular application over the warts should be continued for longer periods to get the desired effect.

Cashewnut Oil: It is extracted from the shells of cashewnuts. It acts on the warts by irritating them.

Onions: Onion piece, when rubbed over the warts, causes some irritation. Used over longer periods, warts disappear, especially if they are small.

Kasisadi Tailam should be applied on the warts for 15 days as an external application.

14. WHITLOW

INTRODUCTION

A pus-filled small abscess or boil on the finger tip, usually next to the nail is called 'whitlow'.

HOME REMEDIES

1. Make a suitable hole in a lemon fruit. Thrust the affected finger inside the lemon for 30 minutes a day for relief.
2. A poultice prepared from rice flour and linseeds (Linium ussitatissimum), when applied on the affected finger gives prompt relief.

METHOD OF PREPARATION

Grind well *alivithu* seeds with lemon juice or cold water and prepare poultice (pastelike) by adding required quantity of rice flour.

AYURVEDIC REMEDIES

Available over the counter for this are *Triphala Guggul*. 2 pills twice a day with water should be taken for 15 days.

Causative Factors

'Whitlows' can be caused by a virus or by a bacterium that enters the body through a cut. People who work in water, like washermen are likely to suffer more.

Signs & Symptoms

- The finger around the nail swells and becomes painful to touch..
- A blister of pus may develop alongside the nail.
- In a more severe infection, the skin around the nail is also affected.
- Fever and sleeplessness occur.

15. PRICKLY HEAT

INTRODUCTION

It is an acute form of rash associated with excessive sweating, especially during humid climate.

TREATMENT

HOME REMEDIES

1. Grapes and its juice should be taken 200ml daily.
2. Plenty of buttermilk should be consumed.

3. *Dhania* is a popular remedy of it. A cold infusion of it is taken 50ml. twice daily.
4. *Dab* (coconut water) should be taken on empty stomach.
5. *Sattu* mixed with water and a pinch of sugar gives immediate relief.

AYURVEDIC REMEDIES

1. *Parval pish* 250mgm is taken twice daily with honey.

For details on Ayurvedic Remedies, refer to Glossary

DO'S & DON'TS

Exposure to fresh air and daily bath helps both in preventing and curing this condition.

Causative Factors
It is mainly caused due to clogging of sweat pores by application of talcum powder, creams, dirt (not bathing regularly and properly) or due to wearing of non-absorbent clothes which prevent evaporation of sweat.

Signs & Symptoms
It consists of small superficial eruptions which look like grain of sand. It affects almost any part of the body. Itching, burning sensation discomfort and sometimes bacterial infections (pus formation) may accompany.

16. RINGWORM

INTRODUCTION

Ringworm is a skin disease due to infection by fungi. Different fungi affect different parts of the body superficially.

TREATMENT

AYURVEDIC REMEDIES

1. *Paradadi Malham* is useful externally.
2. *Arogya vardhini vati* 1 tab. three times a day.
3. Tab. Rakhoplex (Bharat Pharmacy) 1 tab. 3 times a day.
4. Tab. Skinelle (Charak) 1 tab. 3 times a day.
5. Cap. *Neem* taken daily once on empty stomach.

Causative Factors
It is mainly due to lack of hygiene or not wearing clean, dry, absorbent clothes. Caustic soaps, improper drying, humid weather, lack of immunity give rise to ringworm.

Signs & Symptoms
The infection spreads peripherally and heals centrally leaving a ring with a scaly or vesicular border and a central zone of normal skin. These lesions are very itchy and give rise to secondary infections.

DO'S & DON'TS

Always wear clean clothes and take bath daily. Curd and pickles should be avoided.

1. BURNING URINE

INTRODUCTION

While passing urine, some people feel a burning sensation in the urethra. This may be due to various reasons.

Causative Factors

- Urinary tract infection.
- Venereal diseases.
- Enlarged prostate.
- Stone in urinary bladder.
- Concentrated urine (as in summer).
- Obstruction of urinary passage.

Signs & Symptoms

Other symptoms which accompany burning micturition (urination) are passage of pus from urine, bleeding in urine, fever and stoppage of urination.

TREATMENT

HOME REMEDIES

1. Lemon is popularly used. Lemon juice should be given 2-3 times a day mixed with sugar and water.
2. Carrots are also helpful in controlling burning urine.
3. Radish juice 25ml given twice daily.
4. Fresh coconut water given once a day.
5. Sugarcane also can be consumed as much as one can.
6. *Jamun* is also very good. 100gm should be taken daily.

AYURVEDIC REMEDIES

1. *Gokshururadi Guggulu* is the drug of choice. One tablet three times a day.
2. *Chandraprabhavati* is another which is very effective, 1 tab. twice daily.
3. Tab. Ashmol 2 tab. 3 times a day.
4. Tab. Calcury (Charak) 1-2 tab. 3 times a day.
5. Renalka syrup (Himalaya drugs) 2 tsf mixed with half cup of water three times a day for 15 days.

DO'S & DON'TS

1. Hot spices should be avoided.
2. Exposure to sun and heat is to be avoided.
3. Lots of liquids should be consumed.

2. KIDNEY STONES

INTRODUCTION

The formation of stones in the urinary system is a common disorder in many parts of the country. In fact, areas such as Rajasthan, Saurashtra etc., are called "stone-belts".

These stones are made up of the concentrate of substances usually found in urine. These are uric acid, phosphates, calcium, and oxalic acid. The size of the stones may vary from sand/gravel to the size of a bird's egg. These stones are made up of either calcium oxalate or phosphate. The phosphate varieties generally occur due to infections. Most of the stones, i.e., around 90% are composed of calcium as a principle ingredient.

TREATMENT

Silent stones need little or no treatment. Bigger stones are surgically removed.

However, small stones can be dissolved and passed out through urine by the administration of certain home remedies coupled with some Ayurvedic remedies.

HOME REMEDIES

1. Coconut water is a good home remedy for burning urination and scanty urine. Regular intake also flushes out small particles of dissolved stones through urination.
2. Barley water can also be used for this purpose.
3. Water melon: This contains good amount of water, and is also rich in potassium salts. It is a nutritive as well as a safe diuretic to be used in this condition.
4. Onion decoction: Make the decoction by adding water to some bulbs of onion. Sugar should be added to it and taken.

Causative Factors

In a majority of cases, there is no obvious reason why a kidney stone has developed, but there are a few cases in which the cause is clear. For instance, in patients affected with chronic gout, high levels of uric acid are found in the blood, so that the acid crystallises in the kidneys to form stones.

A kidney infection may cause cells to be shed from the kidney lining forming a focus around which a stone may develop.

People who live in hot climates and do not drink enough fluid/water may also end up with stones, because their urine becomes highly concentrated.

Signs & Symptoms

Some kidney stones produce no symptoms at all but are discovered during a routine check-up. These are known as 'silent' stones. If, however, a kidney stone gets into the urinary tract, and blocks off the flow of urine or starts some infection, it can cause intense pain, which demands emergency treatment.

The pain is first felt in the side and thereafter, in the groin and thighs. There will be a frequent desire to pass urine and painful and burning urination occurs. Nauseating sensation or vomitings and fever with chills also occur in some.

5. The decoction prepared with *Kulathi Dal* is very useful.
6. Soda water is also very useful if taken thrice daily after meals.

AYURVEDIC REMEDIES

1. *Gokshura Kada* is a good Ayurvedic remedy. It is an oral liquid, promoting easy urination and relieves burning sensation. It should be taken 3 to 4 times a day in doses of 15ml with equal quantity of water.
2. Patherina tablet is the specific Ayurvedic remedy for stones. 1 tab. twice a day along with a glass of water ensures good relief.
3. Cystone tab. (Himalaya Drugs) 1 to 2 tablets twice daily for 6 to 8 weeks.
4. Calcury tab. (Charak) 1 to 2 tablets twice or thrice daily for 6 to 8 weeks.
5. *Ber Patthar Bhasma* is the drug of choice.
6. *Chander Prabha Vati* is also very useful in burning micturition. 1 tab. twice daily.

For details on Ayurvedic Standard Medicines, refer to Glossary

DO'S & DON'TS

Liquids/fluids should be taken in good quantity. Food which may irritate the urinary system and kidneys like alcohol, pickles, fish, chicken etc., should be avoided.

Other food items to be restricted are peas, soyabeans, beetroot, cauliflower, carrots, almonds and eggs.

DIET

1. Hot water bath and hot fomentation over the back give relief.
2. *Yoga*: Certain *asanas*, which stimulate kidneys can be practised. These are *Pavana Mukta Asana*, *Uttana Padasana*. These are to be done under the guidance of a *Yoga* expert initially.

3. NEPHRITIS (SWELLING OF KIDNEY)

INTRODUCTION

Nephritis refers to inflammation of the kidney. It involves inflammation of different parts of the kidney due to different reasons.

TREATMENT

HOME REMEDIES

1. Juice of radish 250 ml given 2 or 3 times a day.
2. *Triphala* water or powder is also proved good.

AYURVEDIC REMEDIES

1. *Punarnava Mandoor* is the drug of choice 1 tab. three times a day.
2. Tab. Cystone (Himalaya drugs co.) 1 tab. 3 times a day.
3. 1 Neeri tab is also very effective. Doses are as above.

DO'S & DON'TS

1. Patient should not take much of salt.
2. Lots of liquids especially water is to be taken.
3. Fried and sour things to be avoided.

Causative Factors

- Infections of the urinary system.
- Tuberculosis of the kidney.
- Tumours of the kidney.
- Drugs—painkillers, antibiotics.
- Toxic chemicals and heavy metals.
- Metabolic disorders.

Signs & Symptoms

Usual symptoms are:
- Swelling of the face.
- Urine contains protein (albumin).
- Blood pressure increases.
- Nausea or vomiting.
- Headache.
- Abdominal pain.
- Burning urination, increased frequency.
- Fever.
- Backache.

4. BLOOD IN URINE

INTRODUCTION

Presence of blood in the urine is called haematuria.

Causative Factors

It is commonly caused by urinary stones or infection of the kidney or genital region. Some type of bleeding disorders can also give rise to haematuria.

Signs & Symptoms

Besides these symptoms the patient may have pain in the loin or back, fever, bleeding from other sites, vomiting, pus in urine and protein in urine.

TREATMENT

HOME REMEDIES

1. Green banana is used as vegetable.
2. One glass juice of white pumpkin mixed with sugarcane juice should be given everyday.
3. The powder of *amla* ½ tsf twice daily with water.
4. Pomegranate in any form is very useful.

AYURVEDIC REMEDIES

1. *Gokshura* is the drug of choice. The seeds are used as powder and ½-1 tsf of it given twice a day.
2. *Shilajit* 125mg given twice a day.
3. *Chandraprabhavati* 1-2 tab twice daily.

DO'S & DON'TS

Sexual intercourse is to be avoided and patient should take lots of fluids.

5. PROSTATE ENLARGEMENT

INTRODUCTION

Prostate enlargement is the commonest problem in males above 60 years, and is a normal part of the ageing process.

AYURVEDIC TREATMENT

1. Mild cases respond to *Chandraprabhavati* tablets available over the counter. It is an Ayurvedic medicine used 2 pills twice a day with a cup of warm milk.

2. *Shilajit* is also a drug of choice in this condition. 250mg capsules twice a day with a cup of milk resolve the urinary problem.
3. Prostina capsule (Charak) 1 capsule thrice a day after meals taken for 4 to 6 weeks gives much relief.

For details on Ayurvedic Standard Medicines, refer to Glossary

In advanced stage, surgery known as prostatectomy is the answer.

In case the patient is too ill to be operated upon, a permanent catheter may be the only solution.

Causative Factors

The prostate is a male sex gland about the size of a horse chestnut. It is made up of a cluster of little glands which surround the urethra at the point where it leaves the bladder.

During the long years of life, harmless nodules develop in the tissues. These accumulate and gradually enlarge the gland.

The problem arises only when the gland gets so large that it interferes with the urethra. As the gland enlarges, it narrows the diameter of urethra and impedes the flow of urine.

Signs & Symptoms

- The most common symptom is the frequency with which the patient has to urinate two or three times at night as well as constantly during the day.
- It may be difficult to stop urinating once the process is started.
- The stream is narrower and less powerful than before.
- There may be a tendency to dribble urine.
- After urinating, one still has a feeling of incomplete evacuation.
- Straining may cause some blood to appear in the urine.
- As the condition progresses, it can become very painful, cystitis may develop and, in time the flow of urine may be reduced to a few drops at a time or stop altogether —a condition known as retention.

1. DIABETES

INTRODUCTION

Diabetes mellitus affects one in a 100 people. It is a life-long problem. In most cases, however it can be kept under control by daily usage of drugs. Dietics also play a role in the management.

BACKGROUND

Diabetes has been recognised since ancient times and is of particular importance because of its wide prevalance. The name is derived from the sweet taste of urine from patients with this disorder (mellitus = honey) due to the glycosuria resulting from elevated levels of blood glucose. In Ayurveda, it is known as "*Madhu Meha*" i.e., passing honey-like urine.

DEFINITION

Diabetes mellitus is a condition of impaired carbohydrate utilisation caused by an absolute or relative deficiency of insulin.

There are two main types of diabetes: insulin dependent diabetes and non-insulin dependent diabetes.

1. INSULIN DEPENDENT DIABETES

This type occurs when the body produces virtually no insulin. This usually develops in the early teens though it can appear later. It usually develops very quickly, often over a few days. The child or young adult feels increasingly weak, becomes intensely thirsty, and passes large quantities of urine. She/he may lose weight rapidly

---

Causative Factors

Diabetes is caused by a lack of the hormone insulin, which controls the way the body uses sugar. When one consumes bread, cakes, biscuits and other foods containing sugar and starch, the digestive process in the bowel breaks down the sugar and starch into glucose, which is absorbed into the blood stream. Insulin, which is produced in the pancreas, a small organ located just below the stomach, helps the body process the glucose in the blood, so that it can be used to fuel muscle activity and other body functions. After processing, any excess can be stored in the liver as glycogen to be converted later into energy or fat.

In diabetes, the pancreas does not produce enough insulin to allow the glucose in the blood to be used. In some cases, no insulin at all is produced.

Heredity plays an important part in this disease. Nearly one-third of diabetics have a family history of insulin deficiency.

Age can also cause the pancreas to become inefficient. Many of those who develop the disease in later life are over-weight.

because, unable to use or store its glucose, the body draws on its stores of fat or energy. There may also be confusion and sleepiness. Without prompt treatment, the condition can worsen to such an extent that the diabetic may lose consciousness and pass into a coma. The breath may smell of alcohol.

2. NON-INSULIN DEPENDENT DIABETES

It is a milder form resulting when the body produces some insulin but not enough for its requirements. Most people in this group are over 40 years and over-weight.

The initial symptoms of thirst and excessive urine usually come on over a period of months (gradual onset). Other symptoms like tiredness, a feeling of pins and needles and blurred vision may also occur. But it is very rare for the older diabetic to go into a coma.

DIABETICS — CHARACTERISTICS

Diabetics are more prone to suffer from certain types of infection than other people, because sugar encourages the growth of bacteria/fungi and viri.

Common problems that occur are:

Recurrent boils and carbuncles; thrush and itching in the genital regions because of high blood sugar levels in the urine, and the failure of cuts and other injuries to heal.

TREATMENT

HOME REMEDIES

1. INSULIN DEPENDENT DIABETES

Home remedies or herbal drugs are not yet all effective in this condition, i.e., total lack of insulin. Only insulin injections at regular intervals as determined by the specialist should be taken under his direct supervision.

DIETICS

Once on insulin, diabetics must be careful about food/diet. Regular meals throughout the day are a must. If they have an insulin injection and do not eat, the level of glucose in the blood stream will fall dramatically, and they can become the victims of a hypoglycaemic attack.

Insulin dependent diabetics, apart from regular meals, need to be particularly careful about the quantity of sugar and starch that they eat. They need some but not too much. So diabetic diets are prescribed to contain specified amounts of sugar. A special diabetic diet recommended by the National Institute of Nutrition (NIN) Hyderabad is reproduced in the 'THERAPEUTIC DIETS' chapter of this book for the benefit of the diabetics.

Now-a-days simple kits are available for testing and monitoring the level of sugar in the urine and as well as in blood. This way diabetics can keep their own check and get remedial measures. If there is a low level of sugar, they can take little bit of sugar to avoid hypoglycaemia.

2. NON-INSULIN DEPENDENT DIABETES

This type of diabetes known as NIDD type usually improves with a carefully controlled diet to rid them of any excess weight and reduce their sugar and starch intake.

A regular check should be kept on the blood sugar level, and if it settles in the normal range, no further treatment is needed.

In case, if diet alone is not sufficient, one should try some home-remedies before switching over to regular treatment.

HOME REMEDIES

1. *Amla* (Indian gooseberry) fresh juice 10ml and 2 grams pure *haldi* (turmeric) powder well mixed and taken twice a day, effectively maintains the sugar level and imparts many side benefits like strength and vitality.

2. Bitter gourd, popularly known as *karela* possesses the well marked anti-diabetic activity — Ayurveda also recommends the daily use of this vegetable. The active principle of this "plant insulin" is useful in lowering the sugar levels in blood and urine.
   Fresh juice of two *karelas* (approximately 20ml) should be taken on empty stomach in the early morning daily. The regular practice of this gives enormous benefits to the diabetics.

3. Fenugreek: The National Institute of Nutrition, (NIN), Hyderabad, recently found that fenugreek seeds are effective in controlling diabetes. It is found to be effective in lowering the serum cholesterol and triglycerides apart from sugar. Therefore, this item should be added to *chapatis*, and eaten regularly, apprx. 25 gm of fenugreek seeds are needed daily.

4. Black Berry: also known as *kala jamun* is another home remedy for diabetes. It is extensively used in Ayurveda and other systems of medicine — its bark, fruits, seeds are useful. The inner bark of the *jamun* tree is used in the treatment.

5. Unboiled milk mixed with equal quantity of water taken early in the morning on empty stomach gives very good result.

6. Juice of *satavar* mixed with equal quantity of milk taken once daily is very helpful in controlling sugar level in blood.

AYURVEDIC REMEDIES

1. *Jambavasav* an oral liquid prepared from this bark is available in the Ayurvedic stores. 15ml of this liquid with equal quantity of water should be taken twice daily ½ hour after meals. Useful Ayurvedic drugs available in the market are listed in the glossary of Ayurvedic drugs appended.

2. *Pramch Mihir Tailam* is very good for external massage in the abdominal region.
3. *Jambulin* tablets (Unjha) in the dose of 2 tablets twice daily with water or milk cures early cases of diabetes.
4. Diabecon tablets (Himalaya Drugs) in the dose of 1 to 2 tablets twice daily can be given depending upon the patient.
5. Hyponidd tablets (Charak) can also be added to the existing allopathic medicines for diabetes.
6. Glucomap tablets (Maharishi Ayurved) in the dose of 1 to 2 tablets twice or thrice daily is very useful in diabetes.
7. *Madhumeharyog* tablets (Baidyanath) produce good results in the dose of 1 to 2 tablets once or twice a day.

For details on Ayurvedic Standard Medicines, refer to Glossary

DO'S & DON'TS

<u>Dietics</u>: See the special diets recommended in the chapter 'THERAPEUTIC DIETS'.
<u>Exercise</u>: It is a key factor in the management of diabetes. Briskwalks, jogging, light games and swimming are good toners of the body.
<u>Yoga</u>: Suitable *Asanas* are *Bhujangasana, Dhanurasana, Sarvangasana* etc. These should be performed under expert guidance.

2. GOITRE

INTRODUCTION

This refers to enlargement of the thyroid gland resulting in swelling in the front part of the neck.

TREATMENT

HOME REMEDIES

1. Old rice should be used once a day in food.
2. Barley is another home remedy. Barley water can be taken daily twice a day.
3. Cucumber is also good for goitre patients 100gm of it can be consumed daily as salad.

Causative Factors

- Deficiency or increase in iodine content of food items.
- Thyroid tumours.
- Due to medicines.
- Pregnancy.

Signs & Symptoms

These depend on the cause and the type of goitre. The thyroid gland in such cases may be functioning less than normal or more than normal. The goit in many cases due to its large size, may produce problems in speech, respiration and swallowing of food.

AYURVEDIC REMEDIES

1. *Kanchanara Guggulu* is the drug of choice 2-3 tablets three times a day with milk or warm water.
2. *Punarnava Mandoor* and *Guggulu* can also be used side by side. One tab. three times a day.

DO'S & DON'TS

1. Exercise of neck is useful in this condition.
2. Sour and heavy foods are contraindicated.

3. CERVICAL SPONDYLOSIS

INTRODUCTION

A type of arthritis affecting the cervical and the intervertebral discs of the spine, producing pain in the neck ...... region. It is termed as critical spondylosis.

Causative Factors

The main causative factor is the aging of bones and joints. Trauma, incorrect posture of the body, prolonged typing or writing with flexion of the neck aggravate the symptoms.

Signs & Symptoms

Pain in the back of the neck spreading at times to the shoulder, arms and even chest and forehead. The pain is aggravated by the movement of the neck. When this disease becomes chronic in nature, giddiness numbness of hands and even paraplegia can occur.

TREATMENT

HOME REMEDIES

1. *Neem* is very useful in cervical spondylosis. The flowers as well as leaves can be consumed on daily basis.
2. Any oil available at home mixed with camphor *(karpur)* can be used for massage of neck.
3. One string of garlic is to be taken daily on empty stomach.

AYURVEDIC REMEDIES

1. *Singhanada Guggulu* is popularly used. One tab. three times a day with hot water or hot milk for 15-30 days.
2. *Punarnavadi Guggulu* is also used for controlling inflammation. 1 tab. three times a day.
3. Tab. *Pirant* (Maharishi Ayurved) 1 tab 3 times a day.

4. Cap. Arthocare (Uttam) 1 cap. 3 times a day.
5. Tab. Rumalaya (Uttam) 1 tab. 2-3 times a day.
6. *Mahanarayan Taila* is good for massage.
7. *Pirant* oil can also be used for same purpose.

DO'S & DON'TS

1. Wheat is better than rice, *maida* and *suji*.
2. Exposure to cold is avoided.
3. Sour things, particularly curd, etc. are strictly prohibited.

4. BACK-ACHE

INTRODUCTION

Back-ache or pain is one of the most commonly prevalent complaints, more especially in women. Many back pains have no immediately obvious cause.

TYPES OF BACK PAINS

The facet joints linking one vertebra to the next one can also be damaged or strained.

1. Lumbago: A pain in the lower or lumbar region of the back. It is a degenerative problem.
2. Fibrositis: Inflammation of the muscles supporting the back. It is also known as 'trigger point' phenomenon.

| TREATMENT |

HOME REMEDIES

Garlic is the most useful home remedy in back problems. This can be used in many forms internally as well as externally.

Causative Factors

In most cases back-ache is due to :
- Strained ligaments,
- Painful muscle spasm,
- Inflammation caused by bad posture,
- Lifting heavy loads in incorrect way,
- Sudden strain through twisting,
- Inadequate support like poorly crafted seats, work tables or too soft mattresses, or
- Emotional problems.

Signs & Symptoms

- Pain is experienced generally either in the middle of the back or the lower region.
- Pain radiates towards both sides of the waist and the hips.
- In acute stage, the patient is bedridden and unable to move.

EXTERNAL APPLICATION

1. Crush 5 Garlic cloves after removing outer covering, add this to 50ml of *til* oil. Boil it for 20 minutes. Then filter it and apply this oil on the painful back and gently massage for 10 minutes. This can be done twice a day.

INTERNAL USE

1. Crush two garlic cloves (duly removing the outer cover and inner pedicel) and add this to a glass of milk. Boil it on a mild flame till ¼th glass remains. Filter and make two equal parts and take it 1 part in the morning and 1 part in the evening. This should be repeated for 30 days for better results.
2. Pure castor oil is also one of the good home remedies for backache. 5 to 10 ml well mixed in a cup of hot milk should be taken duly at bed time for 40 days. This brings in relief.

AYURVEDIC REMEDIES

1. *Simhanada Guggul* — 2 pills twice a day with warm milk.
2. *Dashamoola Kashayam* — 15ml with equal quantity of lukewarm water twice a day.
3. *Ksheera-bala* oil for massage on the affected areas.
4. *Yograj Guggulu* 1 to 2 tablets thrice daily with warm milk or water.
5. Rumalaya tablet (Himalaya Drugs) 1 to 2 tablets twice daily.
6. *Maharasnadi Kwatham* 15ml with half cup of warm water twice daily.

_____

For details on Ayurvedic Standard Medicines, refer to Glossary

DO'S & DON'TS

1. The person should always sleep on a hard bed and maintain a good posture (with proper back rest) while sitting.
2. When pain is less, *Yogasanas* to strengthen the back muscles and bone give a permanent relief.

5. SCIATICA

INTRODUCTION

Sciatica is one of the very painful conditions, most commonly accompanying back pain. This severe pain shoots along the sciatica nerve, affecting all or part of the buttock, thigh, calf and foot area of one side of the body and rarely of both sides.

TREATMENT

HOME REMEDIES

The best home remedy is bed rest.

1. To ease the pain, tamarind soaked in salt water, churned, filtered and boiled to paste-like consistency should be applied warm to the affected leg.

2. Crush 5 garlic cloves, put this in 50ml of *til* oil, allow it to become lukewarm, and apply on the affected areas of pain.

3. One good home remedy for sciatica is the regular application of castor oil to the sole of the affected side. Oil should be made lukewarm before application. Regular practice of this gives good relief.

AYURVEDIC REMEDIES

1. *Simhanada Guggul* is a good remedy in sciatica. Two pills should be taken twice a day after meals with a cup of warm milk.

2. *Maha Vishagarbha Tailam*, an external oil should be applied over the areas of pain before going to bed daily. An early morning warm water bath reduces the inflammation and pain considerably.

3. *Godanta Mishran* along with *Punarnava Guggulu* is very effective.

4. *Brihat Vat Chintamani Ras* 1 tablet 2 to 3 times daily with *Maharasnadi Kwatham* is very effective in acute cases.

DO'S & DON'TS

DIET: One should avoid potatoes, brinjal, curd and cold water/drinks.

Causative Factors

Pressure on a spinal root of the sciatica nerve often due to a slipped disc, facet joint injury or displacement. It can be brought on by (a) lifting heavy objects, (b) sitting in improper posture etc., (c) any condition that results in pressure on the sciatic nerve, such as a tumour, or abscess in a nearby muscle.

Signs & Symptoms

- Mild to intense pain in the buttock, thigh, calf or foot, or in all these areas is experienced.
- If the pressure is more on the nerve, numbness will also be felt.
- The numbness, however, is not always accompanied by back pain and this can lead to sciatica being mistaken for a pulled muscle.
- If one experiences numbness, a feeling of pins and needles and loss of bladder control along with sciatica, the nerve pressure could be bad enough to cause permanent damage. This requires immediate medical attention.

6. ARTHRITIS

INTRODUCTION

The term 'Arthritis' refers to at least 25 different diseases, the most common being rheumatoid arthritis, osteoarthritis and gouty arthritis. All these are characterised b·· inflammation in one or more joints.

TREATMENT

HOME REMEDIES

1. 10 gm of dry ginger powder (*sonth*) well mixed with 15ml castor oil may be taken internally for relief from painful joints for 40 days continuously.
2. A confection of garlic and *til* oil (2 cloves + 30ml oil) may be taken internally and the oil boiled with garlic may be applied over the painful joints for relief.
3. Heated papaya or *nirgundi* or castor leaves may be applied over the painful areas. Also onion juice with mustard oil may be applied on the affected joints.

AYURVEDIC REMEDIES

1. *Simhanada Guggulu*: It is available in the pill form. 2 pills i.e., 500mg twice a day with lukewarm water should be taken for 40 days for sustained relief. (Since this contains castor-oil, it may in rare cases cause loose motions, which can be controlled by reducing the dose from 2 pills to 1 pill).
2. *Maha Rasnadi Kada*, an oral liquid should be taken along with the above said pills, in the dosage schedule of 20ml with equal quantity of lukewarm water twice a day.
3. *Mahayograj guggulu* can be given with good results. In winters two tablets 3 to 4 times a day and in summers two tablets 2 times a day with warm water or warm milk.
4. *Mahanarayan Tailam* is used for massage.
5. *Brihat Vat Chintamani Ras* is a drug of choice given in the dose of 125mg to 250mg twice or thrice daily.

For details on Ayurvedic Standard Medicines, refer to Glossary

7. OBESITY

INTRODUCTION

The term "obesity" applies when a person has excessive body fat and is at least 20 per cent heavier than he or she should be in proportion to his height and physique. It is a common problem in western countries and in higher income groups of developing nations like India.

TREATMENT

HOME REMEDIES

Regular exercise helps up to a point. Therefore the best approach is to blend dieting and exercise suitably.

A sensibly balanced and slimming diet is the cornerstone in the management of obesity.

Lemon juice and honey: One teaspoonful of honey, and fresh juice of half a lemon should be well mixed and added to a glass of lukewarm water and taken twice or thrice a day.

AYURVEDIC REMEDIES

1. *Triphala* decoction can be prepared by adding 20gm of *Triphalachurna* to 200ml of water and boiled till 50ml remains. After filtering, this oral liquid should be taken twice a day i.e., 25ml morning and 25ml evening along with pills of *Medohara Vidangadi Loha*, an Ayurvedic medicine available over the counter. This combination is effective in the long run.

2. *Arogya Vardhini Vati* in the dose of 1 to 2 tablets twice daily is very effective in controlling obesity.

For details on Ayurvedic Standard Medicines, refer to Glossary

DO'S & DON'TS

DIET: Bread, sugar, refined cereals, meat, fish, fast food, fatty and fried food must be avoided. Intake of salt should also be restricted.

Causative Factors

- Eating errors: Usually obesity is the result of eating too much, allowing more calories into the body than are being used up by energetic exercise.
  Obese peoples' energy requirements may be less because of a slower metabolic rate.
- Inherited factors: A tendency to obesity can be an inherited one, which runs in the family.
- Hormonal factors: Rarely, obesity can develop as a result of hormonal disorders such as hypothyroidism.

Signs & Symptoms

- Obesity is a grave problem as the extra accumulated fat puts a strain on the vital organs like heart, kidney and liver as well as on large weight bearing joints of hips, knees, and ankles.
- Obese persons are susceptible to several critical diseases like coronary thrombosis, heart failure, hypertension, diabetes, arthritis etc.
- Obesity is the hunting ground for diseases.
  To sum up, "The longer the belt, the shorter the life".

1. PRE-MENSTRUAL SYNDROME (PMS)

INTRODUCTION

This is also known as premenstrual tension, a term encompassing the emotional and physical symptoms that affect women in the days leading up to their monthly period.

In depressed women, it manifests in its worst form.

Ayurveda views this painful menstruation as *Rajah Krichhra.*

Lower pelvis in Ayurveda is considered as the main location of *Apanavata,* which is responsible for elimination of menstrual blood, stool, urine, etc. Women having a tendency towards constipation or those who do not develop healthy bowel habits, are usually prone to this type of complaint.

As such Ayurvedic physicians suggest a purgative about two days before the scheduled date of onset of periods.

Causative Factors

- Exact cause is still unknown.
- Many feel that PMS is due to hormonal changes that take place during the period.
- Depression over long periods.

Signs & Symptoms

- Depression & fatigue.
- Aggression and tearfulness.
- Breasts may become tender and feel heavy.
- Bloated tummy.
- Swollen ankles.
- Back-ache, head-ache and pain in the lower abdomen.
- The problems usually occur a few days before bleeding, but they can start upto 2 weeks before and continue during the period itself.

TREATMENT

HOME REMEDIES

1. Crush the leafy pulp of Aloe vera, to express fresh juice. Taking 5 teaspoonful of juice well mixed with 2 tsf of pure honey twice a day for 40 days gives good and long lasting relief from PMS.
2. The cold infusion prepared from lemon grass with the powder of black pepper in dosage schedule of 2 to 4 ozs is effective.
3. Ajwain 5 gm mixed with a small quantity of gur taken with warm water twice or thrice daily gives good relief.

AYURVEDIC REMEDIES

1. *Kumari Asava* — an oral liquid is highly useful in this condition. It contains mainly Aloe vera, and other anti-spasmodic, digestive ingredients. This should be taken in doses of 20-30ml with equal quantity of lukewarm water twice a day. This should be continued for 2 to 3 cycles to get complete and long lasting relief. It is a well tried and safe drug.
2. *Ashokarishta* 20ml with 20ml water taken twice daily after ½ hour of meals for 2 to 3 cycles.
3. M2 tone tablet/syrup (Charak) is an excellent preparation for PMS.
4. Cystone tablet (Himalaya Drugs) is very effective in controlling PMS.

DO'S & DON'TS

1. The last week of menstrual cycle is a crucial one. During this period one should not take anything that causes constipation.
2. Vegetables like potato, brinjal, should be avoided. Garlic should be taken regularly. This checks gas formation.
3. *Avipattikara Churna* 10 grams should be taken with lukewarm water 2 to 3 days before the expected date.

2. PAINFUL PERIODS

INTRODUCTION

Dysmenorrhoea or painful menstruation is a common problem affecting many women, caused by the forceful contraction of the uterus.

TREATMENT

Exercise has a positive effect on the hormonal balance of the body. It is recommended for the younger group.

HOME REMEDIES

1. A purgative for 2 days before the expected date of menstruation is beneficial.
2. *Hing* or asafoetida can be given powdered after frying in *ghee* or butter. 1 tablespoonful should be taken twice a day with a rice bolus followed by a glass of hot water.

Causative Factors

- In the teens and twenties, hormonal secretions increase uterine contraction thereby causing colicky pain.
- In older women, uterine tumours, ovarian cysts and other diseases might be the cause. Constipation may be associated with this type.

Signs & Symptoms

- Pain is often accompanied by nausea, vomiting, diarrhoea, headache, fatigue and nervousness.
- Pain felt in the lower abdomen varies from mild discomfort to intense pain.
- It persists for a day or two.

3. 4-5 cloves of pasted garlic may be consumed thrice a day to relieve pain.
4. Camphor may be rolled into pills and a pill thrice a day may be consumed and a liniment of camphor may be rubbed on the abdomen.
5. 10 grains of powdered sesame seeds 4 times a day may be taken along with a warm hip bath containing a handful of the seeds.

AYURVEDIC REMEDIES

1. *Kumaryasava*: Six tsp with equal quantity of water should be taken twice a day after food, for a month to render periods painless.
2. Cystone tablet (Himalaya) 1 tablet twice or thrice daily.
3. *Rajaparvartini Vati* (Baidyanath) 1 tablet thrice, daily with warm water may be given a week prior to menses.
4. Evecare syrup (Himalaya) 15ml twice daily.

3. IRREGULAR/EXCESSIVE BLEEDING

INTRODUCTION

This is a very common problem seen in women of reproductive age group. These women either have menstruation at irregular intervals or for a prolonged period. This disorder is also termed as Dysfunctional Uterine Bleeding (D.U.B.).

TREATMENT

HOME REMEDIES

1. Pomegranate is a useful remedy. Seven leaves mixed with seven grains of rice crushed together with a small amount of water. The paste is given to the patient twice daily for 30 days.
2. *Amla* is again very useful in controlling bleeding. It is a rich source of vitamin C. It can be given in any form.

Causative Factors

The causes are many. It is mainly due to imbalance of hormones i.e., estrogen and progesterone. Cancer of the uterus, fibroids, tension and bleeding disorders can cause irregular/exessive bleeding.

Signs & Symptoms

Some women complain of pain in the lower abdomen, in the lumbar region and hips before menstruation. Excessive bleeding can lead to weakness, giddiness, headache, breathlessness, palpitations and anaemia.

AYURVEDIC REMEDIES

1. *Ashokarishtha* is drug of choice. 20ml mixed with equal quantity of water given twice a day after meals.
2. *Lodhrasava* is another preparation. Doses are same as above.
3. Tab. Styplen (Himalaya) 1-2 tab. 3 times a day.
4. Cap. Eve Care (Himalaya) 2 cap. twice daily for 30 days then 1 cap. twice daily for 60 days completely cures excessive bleeding.

OTHER MEASURES

1. Exercise should be completely avoided.
2. While sleeping the foot of the bed should be slightly raised.
3. Complete mental and physical rest is suggested.

4. MENOPAUSE

INTRODUCTION

Menopause is a broad term to which the whole range of physical and emotional changes that occur around the time a woman's monthly periods cease, is attributed.

Fertility comes to an end. Usually this change of life happens between the age of 45-50 years, and brings in certain peculiar features.

HEALING HINTS

HOME REMEDIES

1. Milk is a rich source of calcium and vitamin 'D'. Since these get depleted around menopause a good quantity of milk should be given duly in divided doses.

AYURVEDIC REMEDIES

1. Liquorice popularly known as *yasti madhu* or *meethi lakdi* is a natural source of female hormone — oestrogen, and is given in doses of 1 teaspoonful twice a day with warm milk.

Causative Factors

The ovaries stop producing eggs and there is a marked change in hormone levels especially a reduced level of oestrogen.

Signs & Symptoms

In many women, the menopausal change occurs without any unpleasant symptoms, the only change being the cessation of menstrual flow.

However in some others, many disturbing changes take place like:

- Hot flushes and night sweats
- Vaginal dryness
- Increased facial hair
- Dryness of the skin all over the body

Later on, bones can become more brittle. This is called osteoporosis, a condition prone for easy fractures, and the arteries become narrower.

2. *Aswgandha* botanically known as withania somnifera can also be given to calm down irritant behaviour of menopausal women. 5 grams of this powder, well mixed in milk can be given twice a day. It effectively checks the emotional problems associated with menopause.

DO'S & DON'TS

1. Exercises such as jogging, walking, swimming, and cycling are beneficial.
2. One should not indulge in excessive worry and thinking.
3. Women should not worry too much about getting old or losing beauty as these are natural changes.
4. Sound sleep and relaxation are vital to handle this condition.

5. LEUCORRHOEA
(WHITE DISCHARGE)

INTRODUCTION

Normal vaginal discharge should be differentiated from the so-called white discharge. Just as the degree of sweating differs in various people, the degree of vaginal discharge also differs considerably in various women. Most women do not know these variations, and a number of ailments like backache, weakness, joint pains and all ill-health in general are often attributed by them to the so-called 'white discharge'. Some doctors are also inclined to endorse their thinking.

TREATMENT

HOME REMEDIES

1. A warm vaginal douche with *Triphala* water is highly beneficial. Take 20 grams of *Triphala* powder, add to 2 litres of water and boil for 15 minutes—filter it and use as douche, when it is tolerably hot.

Causative Factors

The common local causes of leucorrhoea are:
- Trichomonal vaginitis
- Monilial vaginitis and
- Cervicitis

Signs & Symptoms

Trichomonal Vaginitis: It is the most local cause of leucorrhoea with a history of yellowish and frothy discharge, and the presence of itching locally more or less confirms this. Sometimes, the husband of the patient also develops itching of the penis after a sexual intercourse.

Monilial Vaginitis: This occurs in any case of leucorrhoea where the patient is a diabetic or is pregnant or is receiving antibiotics or oral contraceptive pills.

Cervicitis: This is the third most common local cause of leucorrhoea, with associated problems like back pain.

2. Cold hip bath : Similarly a cold hip bath twice a day is also useful in removing the morbid matter.
3. Fenugreek seeds: These are useful when a tea like decoction is made from these seeds and taken internally.
4. *Tandulodaka* (rice-wash) is very useful for douching.
5. The decoction of bark of *Lodhra* is also used for the purpose of douching.

AYURVEDIC REMEDIES

1. *Pushyanuga Churna*—a powdered medicine is highly useful in leucorrhoea— 3 grams of this powder should be taken twice a day with a cup of milk or rice wash.
2. *Ashokarishta* is also effective. This oral liquid can be taken internally in the dosage form of 20ml+20ml water, twice a day along with *Pushyanuga Churna*.
3. Lukol tablet (Himalaya Drugs) 1 to 2 tablets twice daily.
4. Femiforte tablet (Charak) 1 tablet twice daily.
5. Femiplex tablet (Charak) 1 tablet thrice daily.
6. V-gel (Himalaya Drugs) is the only drug available for external application in the dose of 5gm twice daily for 14 days. Abstinence should be maintained.

OTHER MEASURES

Diet: Non-vegetarian diet like fish, chicken, eggs should be avoided for some days. Instead fresh greeny vegetables, milk, and ghee should be taken more.

6. INFERTILITY

INTRODUCTION

Infertility is the inability in a woman to conceive or in a man to induce conception. It is a problem of grave concern for childless couples, who feel that life is void without a child.

TREATMENT

Sperm and egg production can sometimes be improved with medicines. Tubal obstructions can be dealt with by surgery.

Causative Factors

Infertility can be due to factors affecting one or both the partners.
● The man's sperms have to be healthy, in sufficient numbers and finally they need to be deposited high enough in the woman's vagina to make their way to an ovum.

If there is trouble with conception, it could be because:

Contd ...

HOME REMEDIES

1. Banyan Tree Bark: The bark of this tree should be removed and dried well in the shade. Then this bark should be finally powdered. 10 gm of this powder along with 10 gm of sugar should be taken once early in the morning by both the partners daily for 60 days. This may help in this condition.
2. The root of *Lakshmana* taken during *Pushya Nakshatra* and crushed in *gheekavar* juice and then taken orally. It is to be taken with milk mixed in pure *ghee* on empty stomach for 3 to 7 days after menses.

AYURVEDIC REMEDIES

1. *Phala Ghritam* is an ideal medicine in female sterility if the damage is purely functional and not structural. 5 gm of this medicated ghee should be taken well mixed in a cup of hot milk once a day in the morning.
2. *Aswagandha* powder 5 gm once a day with milk is the good remedy for male partners.
3. *Vanga Bhasma* is a drug of choice given in the dose of 120mg mixed with honey twice daily.
4. M2 tone syrup (Charak Pharma) 2 teaspoons mixed with equal quantity of water taken twice daily after meals for 2 to 3 cycles.
5. Addyzoa tablet (Charak) 2 tablets twice daily with water or milk is very effective in male infertility.
6. Speman Forte and Tentess Forte tablets of Himalaya drugs are both useful drugs for males.

a) The man's sperm count is low, or
b) Because there is a blockage in his spermatic tubes.
● Similarly in the woman's case:
a) She may not be producing eggs
b) Her Fallopian tubes may be blocked
c) Sometimes her womb can be retroverted (tipped backwards) or filled with fibroids
d) Her cervical mucous can be hostile to sperms

Apart from these there are many other reasons why conception does not take place, including the fact that the couple may not be indulging in sexual intercourse around the time of ovulation.

Signs & Symptoms

If a couple have had normal, regular intercourse without using contraception for a year and the woman has not conceived, then the chances are that there is a fertility problem and they should consult a doctor, who may refer them to a fertility centre.

DO'S & DON'TS

The female partner should keep the lower part of her body in a raised position, during sexual act, and for 15 minutes after the act. This allows the sperms to be deposited higher up in the genital tract.

7. FRIGIDITY

INTRODUCTION

The term 'frigidity' is generally used to describe a long term lack of sexual drive and response. It can affect both sexes but is more usually applied to women.

TREATMENT

Blindly trying to do better in bed is less useful than improving the basic relationship. So, talk with your partner about all your problems, hopes and fears, and try to solve them together.

Still, if one finds it hard to communicate, it is better to consult a doctor and trained counsellor.

AYURVEDIC REMEDIES

1. *Ashwagandha Lehyam* is the drug prescribed in this condition. It is a good anti-stressor, nervine and sex tonic, useful for both the partners. Regular use promotes sexual interest in both the partners. Teaspoonfuls of this semi-solid medicine should be taken twice a day with a cup of warm milk. This should be taken for 40 days continuously.
2. *Trasina* capsule (Gufic Laboratories) 1 capsule twice daily with water or milk after meals for a month controls frigidity.
3. *Aagosh* capsule (Platinum Remedies) in the dose of 1 capsule twice daily taken with warm milk after meals for 6 weeks is a good remedy for frigidity.
4. Aswal Plus Capsule (Gufic Pharma) 1 capsule once daily produces desired results in 4 to 6 weeks.
5. Adbac capsule (Uttam) 1 capsule once daily is very useful in improving the stamina thus helping in controlling frigidity.

DO'S & DON'TS

A good nutritive as well as tasty diet gives wonderful results in frigidity.

Causative Factors

Anxiety about performance is a major turn-off when it comes to sex. Nearly everyone has occasional worries, but these can become exaggerated when one places too much emphasis on the physical, as opposed to the emotional side of love-making.

Conflict within the relationship is another important factor. If a couple is always arguing or one partner is resentful of the other, it can lead to problems in bed.

Equally, if one is very tired or worried about other things in life, it can affect libido. Other causes of frigidity include having been sexually abused as a child, over dependence on parents, depression, fear of pregnancy, and other health problems such as multiple sclerosis, and diabetes.

Signs & Symptoms

Sex drive varies from person to person and fluctuates for all types of reasons.

A serious lack of response is indicated when one continuously avoids love making or cannot enjoy it even though the partner is sexually attractive.

8. ANAEMIA

INTRODUCTION

Actually, "an-aemia" means "without blood", but it is generally used to describe people who do not have enough healthy red blood cells in their blood stream. There are many types of anaemia, but in India, mostly in women, the cause of anaemia is commonly iron deficiency and almost 20% of Indian women suffer from it.

TREATMENT

HOME REMEDIES

Adjusting diet is the correct remedy. Eat a nutritious and well balanced diet. Meat, especially kidney and liver and all dairy products are rich in Iron and Vitamin B_{12}. Folic acid is found in green vegetables.

AYURVEDIC REMEDIES

1. *Punarnava Mandoora*, readymade Ayurvedic pills are to be given orally, 1 pill twice a day with a glass of milk. It improves blood condition by increasing haemoglobin levels and thereby RBC count. It is effective even in conditions of oedema due to anaemia.
2. *Lohasavam* is an oral liquid containing iron and other essential factors required for proper production of RBC. 15ml of the tonic should be mixed with 15ml of lukewarm water and consumed twice a day after meals.
3. *Raktda* tablet (Maharishi Ayurved) one tablet once or twice daily for 6 weeks is very useful in anaemia.
4. *Navayas Loh* 120mg taken twice daily is a very good Ayurvedic preparation.
5. *Triphala* powder ½ to 1 teaspoonful twice a day is also very good.

For details on Ayurvedic Standard Medicines, refer to Glossary

Causative Factors

Bleeding such as heavy periods in women is the main cause. The condition may also be due to the excessive destruction of red blood cells so that the bone marrow cannot produce enough to replace those that are lost. Another cause could be insufficient production of RBCs due to a number of factors.

Iron deficiency anaemia is caused by a shortage of iron, a vital component for RBC production. Vitamin deficiency anaemia and pernicious anaemia are both forms of anaemia in which there is inadequate supply of vitamin B_{12} and folic acid.

Signs & Symptoms

Anaemics feel particularly tired because the body is not getting enough oxygen for its routine needs. The skin tends to lose its healthy bloom, and the face becomes pale. If the condition becomes severe, the person will also be short of breath and the ankles may swell.

DO'S & DON'TS

DIET

Sour things, like curd and fried items should be avoided as far as possible. Green vegetables are rich in iron and folic acid and as such these should be taken in plenty. *Til* seeds and jaggery should be taken regularly as these are rich in iron.

If constipation occurs, *Triphalachurna* in a dose of 5 grams should be taken with lukewarm water at bed time.

All these measures, if taken properly, can successfully treat mild to moderate anaemia at home itself.

1. IMPOTENCE

INTRODUCTION

Sex is a part of productive life, and like hunger, is also a basic instinct. In some males, this 'act' becomes difficult to perform.

Impotence is the failure of a man to achieve or maintain an erection, and is more common in older men. Sometimes this term 'impotence' is also used when a man can have an erection but cannot ejaculate semen.

TREATMENT

REASSURANCE: A sympathetic partner can contribute a lot in helping a man overcome this problem. Similarly the man should assure his partner that he still very much wants to show and receive affection.

Despite all these, if a couple cannot work it out together, it is worth consulting a doctor.

If a physical cause is found, suitable medical treatment should be taken.

HOME REMEDIES

1. Garlic: Garlic is a powerful aphrodisiac and regular use keeps a man fit and fertile. In Ayurvedic medicine it has been described as poor man's nectar. It works wonderfully in all types of impotence, resulting from over-indulgence and nervous exhaustion.
   5 to 6 garlic cloves should be crushed having removed the outer coverings and added to a glass of milk, boiled and reduced to ½ glass. Then it should be filtered, required sugar

Causative Factors

Psychological

The most common reason for a man failing to get an erection is psychological. He might be overtired, overstressed, worried or just desperately lacking self-confidence, or it may be due to excessive demands or criticism of his performance by his partner.

Any type of hostility, anger or resentment towards his partner, constant fear of making a woman pregnant, guilt perhaps about an affair or any other negative feeling about sex, can also be the factors.

Physical

Sometimes 'impotence' can be traced back to certain health problems like diabetes, severe depression, or severe reaction to any drug. Excessive alcohol drinking or cigarette smoking can also lead to impotence.

Signs & Symptoms

There are varied types of impotence:
- If failing to get an erection is a rare and short-lived problem, it is normal.
- But when it becomes a long drawn problem after a period of normal sexual function, it has to be attended to urgently.

Contd ...

should be added and taken twice a day in
two equal doses.

2. Dried dates also produce aphrodisiac action.
These should be taken daily as a supplement.
3. Black raisins are also useful.

> • There are a few men who right
> from young age have difficulty
> in achieving an erection enough
> to sustain intercourse.

AYURVEDIC REMEDIES

1. *Ashwagandha Lehyam* is the common medicine for this disorder. It should be taken internally in the dosage of 10 to 15 gm twice a day with a cup of warm milk.
2. *Musli Pakam* taken 2.5 to 5gm once or twice daily with warm milk gives good results.
3. *Ashwagandharishta* 1 to 2 ounces twice daily after meals with equal quantity of water is a useful remedy.
4. *Kapikacchu* is a drug of choice but should be taken under medical supervision.

   There are many other powerful medicines in Ayurveda for the treatment of impotence. These are to be taken under Ayurvedic physician's supervision, as such they are not listed here.

DO'S & DON'TS

Massage: An energetic massage all over the body is highly useful in this condition. *Sri Gopala Tailam*, an Ayurvedic medicated oil should be applied over the hip and pelvic region, before massage.

Yoga: Certain *yogasanas* like *sarvangasana* and *dhanurasana* are indicated.

2. PREMATURE EJACULATION

INTRODUCTION

Premature ejaculation is a condition in which a man passes out semen either before or soon after entering his female partner during sexual intercourse.

This is a common phenomenon occuring in most men at some point or other, but is more common in very young men and can have a demoralising effect on both partners.

TREATMENT

Reassurance is the best treatment.

1. It is a passing problem, and in most cases, is resolved in due course of time.
2. One should just try to forget about it and even laugh it off. This can do wonders.
3. If it becomes a long term problem, seek a doctor's opinion. He may suggest sexual counselling.

AYURVEDIC REMEDIES

Ayurvedic system of medicine offers a wider line of treatment covering psychosomatic-sexual axis. There are rich and highly effective drugs

Causative Factors

● The chief causative factor in many instances - man is worried about how he is likely to perform.
● Man tries to make love too hurriedly.
● Psychological causes, like stress, emotion also play a role.

Signs & Symptoms

Ejaculating before or very soon after penetration is the main symptom, causing embarrassment to both the partners.

available which should be used under supervision of an Ayurvedic Physician. These are known as *Stambhaka* drug measures which delay ejaculation.

1. *Ashwagandha Churna* in doses of 5gms twice a day with milk helps in this condition.
2. *Jatiphala* (Myristica Fragrans) pasted with milk is also an effective remedy, when used in doses of 3-5 gms twice a day.
3. Speman tablet (Himalaya Drugs) 1 to 2 tablets taken twice a day after meals, is a useful remedy for premature ejaculation.
4. Tentex Forte tablet (Himalaya Drugs) in the above doses is another useful treatment for premature ejaculation.

1. BED-WETTING

INTRODUCTION

Bed-wetting means involuntary urination in bed at night. Children generally after the age of 3-4 years gain control over the bladder, but in some children, this mechanism somehow is not strengthened and they pass urine in bed involuntarily. This phenomenon continues even upto 15-20 years of age, putting the teenagers in an embarrassing situation. Boys outnumber girls in this problem.

Causative Factors

'Bed-wetting' can happen due to physical and emotional causative factors. Infection in the urinary system i.e., in the bladder or kidney or a structural defect in the tract, or sometimes thread worms in the stool may also cause the problem.

The psychological factors involved are emotional immaturity, shyness, conflicts between parents, fear, rivalry among children, problem of adjustment in school and feeling of insecurity.

Signs & Symptoms

Involuntary urination in bed at night.

TREATMENT

HOME REMEDIES

1. A teaspoonful of pure honey should be given to the child before going to bed.
2. *Sarshapa* i.e., *Sarson* powder, well mixed in a cup of milk, if given at night before going to bed, stops the wetting.

AYURVEDIC REMEDIES

1. *Shilajitvadi Vati* ½ tablet twice a day with some warm milk usually gives good results.
2. *Chandraprabha Vati* is also a good remedy in this condition. ½ tablet twice a day is given.
3. Neo tablet (Charak) in the dose of 1 to 2 tablets twice daily for two to three months gives good results.

For details on Ayurvedic Standard Medicines, refer to Glossary

DO'S & DON'TS

1. The child/teenager should not be scolded in the evening or before going to bed.

2. He should be asked to urinate before going to bed.
3. Oral liquids like milk, water etc., should be restricted after 4 p.m.
4. Food items like potato, spicy food, etc., should not be given, as these cause gas formation.
5. Evening walks should be encouraged.

2. MEASLES

INTRODUCTION

Measles is a viral disease usually occurring in children. It is considered one of the most contagious of all infections. One attack usually gives immunity for life.

TREATMENT

HOME REMEDIES

Turmeric, *neem*, lemon, and *tulsi* are the well-known remedies for measles.

1. These can be used internally as well as externally on the rashes.
2. A combination of pure turmeric powder 2 gms well mixed in 20ml of fresh juice of *tulsi* leaves, consumed twice a day till the symptoms are cleared, is a valuable remedy.
3. Fresh *neem* leaves well pounded with some turmeric and sandalwood can be used as external paste.
4. If there is persistent cough, *tulsi* juice well mixed with honey can be given repeatedly.

Causative Factors

It is caused by a virus which is spread through the air by coughing and sneezing. People can spread the infection to others as early as a day after making contact with the disease and remain infectious for about a week after the symptoms first appear.

Signs & Symptoms

Symptoms appear 7 to 14 days after exposure to the virus. These usually start with a fever, running nose, sore eyes and a feeling of weakness.

A cough and sore throat soon follow. After a few days, a rash with small rounded spots appears on the sides of the face and the neck, and gradually spreads throughout the body surfaces. With time these spots turn darker from pink colour.

AYURVEDIC REMEDIES

1. Liquorice powder 2gms along with 10ml of honey is also a good remedy to relieve sore throat and cough in measles.
2. *Brihat Haridra Khanda* granules should be taken in a dosage of 5gm well mixed in a cup of lukewarm water twice a day.
3. *Tribhuvan Kirti Ras* in the dose of 1 tablet thrice daily with warm water.

4. *Mahalaxmi Vilas Ras* ½ tablet thrice daily.
5. *Swarn Makshik Bhasma* is a drug of choice in the dose of 125mg thrice daily.

For details on Ayurvedic Standard Medicines, refer to Glossary

DO'S & DON'TS

The affected child should be placed in a clean well ventilated environment. Liquid diet consisting of milk and fresh fruit juices should be given initially. Children suffering from measles should be isolated so as to contain the infection. Children should be vaccinated against measles at the advocated time.

3. MUMPS

INTRODUCTION

Mumps refers to an acute infection of the parotid gland near the ears characterized by swelling and other symptoms.

TREATMENT

HOME REMEDIES

1. Garlic—4-5 strings of garlic made into paste and taken twice with milk.
2. The juice of ginger one teaspoonful mixed with honey taken 2-3 times a day.
3. Black pepper ¼ - ½ taken with warm milk twice a day for 7-10 days.

AYURVEDIC REMEDIES

1. *Luxumi Vilas Ras* is a drug of choice. 1 tab. 3 times a day for 7 to 10 days.
2. *Daru Haridra* is commonly used for this disease. The powder of it 1 tsf mixed with honey and *ghee* is applied on affected part preferably at bed time.

For details on Ayurvedic Standard Medicines, refer to Glossary

DO'S & DON'TS

1. Patient should stop taking hot solid food.
2. Neck and head should be kept warm.

1. DEHYDRATION

INTRODUCTION

Dehydration, in simple words, is shortage of water in the body.

| TREATMENT |

HOME REMEDIES

In mild cases of dehydration, the treatment is following the simple thumb rule of replacing the lost fluid. Non-alcoholic drinks may be given in plenty. Coconut water, barley water, sugarcane juice or glucose-water are the best. Nowadays oral rehydration sachets are freely available. They are easy to use, when duly mixed as per the instructions laid down on the cover. Alternatively, one can use a home made rehydrating solution containing a pinch each of sugar and salt in a cup of water.

In severe cases of dehydration, intravenous fluids are essential, and immediate hospitalisation is a must.

Further, dehydration being more serious in children, medical advice is very essential in such cases.

Causative Factors

Dehydration can happen due to:
- Insufficient water/liquid intake or
- Excessive loss of liquids due to diarrhoea, sunstroke or vomitings.

Signs & Symptoms

- Furious thirst.
- Dizziness, nausea (vomiting sensation.)
- Extreme exhaustion.
- Loss of elasticity of skin and wrinkling.

AYURVEDIC REMEDIES

Shadanga Paneeyam, an oral liquid, 20ml + 50ml water should be given as required orally. It is cooling and rehydrative.

2. FEVER

INTRODUCTION

Raised body temperature is known as fever. In medical terms it is called 'Pyrexia'. Many a times fever is a symptom of many diseases.

TREATMENT

A doctor's consultation is a must to know the exact diagnosis on the type of the fever, especially in cases of children, as they may develop convulsions. However some simple remedies are enumerated below, which can be used in mild cases.

HOME REMEDIES

1. *Tulsi* (Holy Basil) is a well known home remedy useful in all types of fevers like viral, bacterial or malarial.
   A decoction can be prepared by adding 10gm of fresh leaves and 2gm of black pepper powder to 50ml of water. This can be taken 3 times a day. It is a good remedy for fevers.
2. *Neem*: Juice of tender fresh leaves of *neem* is also effective in fevers. 1 teaspoonful of the juice well mixed in 2 spoons of honey should be taken twice a day. It works both as curative as well as preventive.

AYURVEDIC REMEDIES

1. *Sudarshana Ghana Vati* 2 tablets thrice a day with black tea should be taken for 7 days.
2. *Amrutharishta*, an oral liquid in a dose of 15ml thrice a day with equal quantity of water is also useful.
3. *Godanti Mishran* 1 to 2 tablets thrice daily reduces fever and pain.
4. *Anand Bhairav Ras* and *Tribhuvan Kirti Ras* are also very effective in fever but should be taken under the supervision of an Ayurvedic physician.

Causative Factors

The normal body temperature is 37° C (98.4° F) but may vary slightly from individual to individual. It also varies half a degree or so throughout the day, and is usually at its lowest in the morning. The minimum body temperature occurs between 2 AM and 7 AM and the maximum occurs between 4PM and 6PM of the day.

- In very hot weather, the body temperature may rise a little more.
- Usually a rise in temperature of a degree or more is caused by some form of infection.

Signs & Symptoms

- A temperature over 37.4° C or 99.4° F may be considered as fever.
- The person's face will probably be flushed, the eyes may be glazed, the body hot to the touch. The person may either feel hot or cold depending on the rise and fall of temperature.
- When the temperature is dropping, the body often sweats profusely.

For details on Ayurvedic Standard Medicines, refer to Glossary

DO'S & DON'TS

1. Cold sponging if the temperature is too high.
2. Easily digestible liquid diet is good.

3. MALARIA

INTRODUCTION

Malaria is a common fever, occurring frequently in tropical regions like India, Africa etc. It often causes severe debility, and anaemia in the victims.

Causative Factors

Malaria is caused by a tiny, single-celled parasite. It is transmitted by the bite of an infected mosquito. The malarial parasites belong to the genus of Plasmodium. The most dangerous member of this family is Plasmodium falciparum.

Signs & Symptoms

- Malaria usually occurs with flu-like symptoms, including a severe headache, body aches, and pains in the muscles.
- Shivering and high temperature. The shivers usually take the form of full blown rigors.
- Temperature rise is dramatic, and vomiting may occur.
- This is followed by a phase of heavy sweating and a fall in temperature.

These cycles of fever may come and go.

TREATMENT

HOME REMEDIES

1. *Tulsi*: The tender leaves of holy basil are the best anti-malarial remedy. Fresh juice extracted from 10 leaves (about 10ml) well mixed with 10ml of honey should be repeated 4 times a day.
2. *Chirayata*: Botanically known as Swertia Chirata, it is a proven remedy for malaria. An infusion is prepared and given.
3. Black tea prepared with *sonth* and black pepper is also useful in the malarial fevers.

AYURVEDIC REMEDIES

1. *Ayush* tablets are proven anti-malarials. 2 tablets thrice a day with hot water is the dose.
   These are available in the market under brand names like Chirakin, Antimal etc.
2. *Sudarshana Ghanavati* is the classical remedy given in doses of 2 tabs. thrice a day.
3. *Amrutarishta* an oral liquid should be given in dose of 30ml with equal quantity of lukewarm water thrice a day. This prevents the debility, that generally occurs.

4. *Godanti Mishran* given in the dose of 125mg three to four times a day.

5. *Shetbhanji Ras* is a drug of choice in the dose of 250mg with honey thrice daily.

For details on Ayurvedic Standard Medicines, refer to Glossary

DO'S & DON'TS

PREVENTION

Malaria can be prevented by protecting from mosquito bites. Hygienic and sanitary conditions should be improved, so as to ensure that there is no pool of stagnant water, where mosquitoes breed.

1. Hydrotherapy should be done to reduce fever.
2. Patient should be adequately covered in case of rigor.
3. Fruit juice of apple, orange, *malta, narangi* should be given.

4. FILARIA

INTRODUCTION

Filariasis or Filaria is caused by the bite of an infected mosquito belonging to the species called Culex.

TREATMENT

HOME REMEDIES

1. Leaves of *bel* tree are very useful in the treatment of this condition. Three leaves everyday help in cure and prevention of this condition.
2. 10 cloves of garlic should be given everyday if patient can tolerate its smell.
3. Dried ginger is used in boiling water.

AYURVEDIC REMEDIES

Nityananda Rasa is very commonly used for it. ½ tab. to 1 tab. two times a day on empty stomach for 2 months.

Causative Factors

The adult worms live in the lymphatic vessels and the females produce microfilariae which at night circulate in the blood. The mosquitoes on biting the infected individuals carry the microfilariae which develop into adult worms. If the same mosquito bites a healthy person, the worms are transmitted to him and the infection is spread.

Signs & Symptoms

The early symptoms are fever accompanied by pain and redness along the affected lymphatic vessels. The testes are affected and swelling and pain occur. In later stages all the lymphatic channels in the lower limbs are affected and legs become swollen giving rise to elephantiasis. Some patients develop urticaria and pneumonia.

1. To prevent mosquito bite, nets should be used regularly.
2. Patient should avoid residing in marshy areas.
3. Hot water must be used for bathing and drinking.

5. AIDS/HIV POSITIVE

INTRODUCTION

Acquired Immuno Deficiency Syndrome, popularly known as 'AIDS', is one of the unforgettable diseases of the 20th century, the black shadows of which may continue into the 21st century also. "Acquired" refers to any condition that is not present at birth. "Immuno Deficiency" means the body's immune (defence) system which is not working efficiently. And 'syndrome' refers to the fact that it includes a group or a range of symptoms and signs. This deficiency is a late consequence of infection by the human immuno deficiency virus (HIV).

HINTS

Follow safe sex practices.

Avoid blood transfusions as far as possible.

Insist on disposable syringes & needles while taking injections.

Causative Factors
High-risk activities that are able to transmit HIV from one person to another include sexual contact - especially unprotected vaginal and anal intercourse and sharing needles and syringes.
However, HIV is not transmitted by insect bites, nor through kissing, coughing, sneezing or sharing a toilet!

Signs & Symptoms
There are many opportunistic infections which may infect the individual and symptoms and signs manifest depending on the system or systems involved and the symptoms are varied and numerous. They include fevers, sweats, cough, diarrhoea, herpes infection, dry itchy skin etc.

TREATMENT

HOME REMEDIES

Persons with AIDS or HIV+ can expect progress in therapy in the near future.

However some antiviral herbs, which strengthen the inner defence system of the body are given below.

HERBAL PROTECTIVES

Daily intake of some herbs for very long periods, may be helpful for some HIV+ people in slowing down the onset of AIDS, just like AZT, a costly drug. These wonder home remedies are two holy plants *tulsi*, *bilva* (*bael* fruit) and one common bulb popularly known as the "heal-all" bulb i.e., garlic. All these are well known antiviral agents and rejuvenatives.

1. *Tulsi* (Ocimum sanctum): A tsf of juice extracted from tender leaves should be taken daily on empty stomach early in the morning. This strengthens the entire respiratory system, generally targeted by HIV.

2. *Bel* fruit (Aegle marmelos): Specially found in holy places like temples, the fruits are highly useful especially the half-ripe fruit. The fruit pulp should be dried and powdered. 1 tsf of the powder along with some water should be taken after meals. This protects the digestive system from invasion by HIV.

3. Garlic *(Lahsun)* (Allium sativum): One piece of a garlic bulb should be taken and the outer layers and inner pedicel removed. It should then be crushed and added to a glass of pure milk. The milk should be boiled on moderate fire till the milk is reduced to ¼ glass. This should be taken with little bit of sugar at bed time daily. This is a wonder rejuvenative and builds up the body mass and weight and is a good anti-viral.

ONION: To treat wrinkles, wash eyes or face in onion juice. Mixed with honey, it acts as a natural antibacterial and antiseptic lotion.

ORANGE PEEL: Dried and ground orange peel is used in a mask and facial scrubs.

ROSE: This highly fragrant flower is the richest source of natural vitamin E or Youth vitamin. Ayurveda recommends Roja Pushpa, deckling a semi-solid (like *gulkand*) to maintain youthfulness. This quenches thirst in summer and combats *... Gulkand* a sweet pan ingredient is made out of rose petals. This cools the overworked brain tissue.

STRAWBERRY: Being a rich source of iron, strawberry juice helps cleaning discoloured teeth when used regularly.

SUGAR, SOAP AND LEMON: For an abrasive face scrub, lather the face with soap then add a handful of sugar and scrub. Rinse off and finally apply lemon juice. This process thoroughly cleanses and stimulates the skin.

TEA: Due to its tannin content, it is soothing and healing as it absorbs ultra-violet light. It is used in sun-tan creams to prevent burning. Teabags also make soothing eye pads.

SKIN AND VITAMINS

* VITAMIN A helps keep skin from drying out by helping circulation.
* VITAMIN B helps keep skin blemish-free.
* VITAMIN C purifies blood and helps keep you glowing. *Amla* and other citrus fruits are full of minerals and vitamin C.
* VITAMIN E is the youthful vitamin helping keep skin young.
* Ample fresh fruits and vegetables, plenty of water and good, sound sleep provide natural nourishment to skin.

HERBALS IN SKIN CARE

* *SHATAVARI* (Asparagus racemoses) is one of the highly useful herbal drugs in skin care. The powder of the root 1 gm in quantity is taken orally with a cup of milk every evening to nourish dry skin and add lustre.
* SILK COTTON TREE: A paste made from the thorny skin of the silk cotton tree with milk and applied removes black spots and brings lustre to the face.
* FENUGREEK SEEDS (*METHI*): The powder applied to the skin prevents dryness, roughness and coarseness.
* COTTON SEED OIL: It is a very useful dressing in clearing spots and freckles on the skin.
* NUTMEG: The local application of nutmeg paste (*jaiphala*) clears out white patches and blemishes on the skin.
* CITRON AND COTUS: A mixture of honey and the juice of citron (*bijora*) in which costus (*kushta*) has been sealed for a week is a useful cosmetic to keep skin soft.

Part-II
Kitchen Remedies

KITCHEN REMEDIES

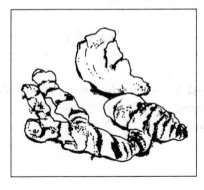

HALDI

1. **HALDI**—*Curcuma longa, Zingiberaceae*
   English   - Turmeric
   Hindi   - Haldi

Chief Actions :-

Stimulant   Carminative
Blood purifier   Antiseptic
Wound healing agent

Applications :-

Internal :-

1. ½ tsp powdered turmeric taken thrice a day relieves flatulence and loss of appetite.
2. 10-20 ml of extracted juice may be taken daily in skin diseases, diabetes and jaundice.
3. ½ tsp each of turmeric along with *Amla* powder should be taken daily early in the morning in diabetes.

External :-

1. In sprains & bruises, a hot paste with lime juice and salt petre is applied.
2. In small pox & chicken pox, a coating is applied to facilitate scabbing.
3. In painful and protruding piles, an ointment along with onions and warm linseed oil gives great relief.
4. Powder of turmeric is sprinkled on wounds/ulcers for speedy healing.
5. In nasal catarrh & coryza, fumes of turmeric powder and over-burnt charcoal may be inhaled for prompt relief. This may be adopted even in common colds.
6. In scorpion bite, the bitten area is exposed to the same fumes for a few minutes to minimise toxicity.

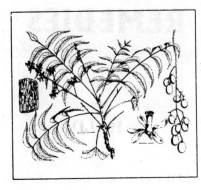

NEEM

2. NEEM — *Azadirachta indica, Meliaceae*
English   -   Margosa tree
Hindi   -   Neem

Chief Actions :-
Antiseptic
Anthelmentic
Astringent

Applications :-
Internal :-
1. The fruit pulp may be used in infestations of worms, in a dose of 5 gm on empty stomach with lukewarm water daily.
2. In indigestion, an infusion of the flowers may be taken in 3 divided doses. 5 gm of neem flowers should be soaked in a glass of water overnight for this purpose.
3. The fruit acts as a purgative in worm infestations.
4. The resin of the tree is used to treat viral infections along with other drugs.

External :-
1. The seed oil is used as an external stimulant in leprosy, urticaria, eczema, scrofula & other skin diseases.
2. A paste of the leaves may be applied on any itching condition of the skin, and on wounds.
3. The leaves are used as a prophylactic against malaria and chicken pox.
4. The decoction of the leaves may be poured as a stream over wounds and ulcers to relieve burning sensation and for fast healing.

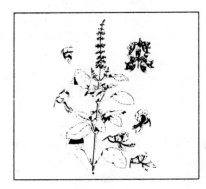

TULSI

3. TULSI—*Ocimum sanctum, Labiatae*
English   -   Holy basil
Hindi   -   Tulsi

Chief Actions :-

Expectorant   Stomachic
Antiviral   Antifungal
Blood purifier

Applications :-

Internal :-
1. Decoction or fresh juice of the leaves may be taken in malaria, bronchitis and nasal catarrh.
   Dose :- One tsf of fresh juice with equal quantity of honey is a sure remedy, when used for 7 days.
2. As an expectorant in wet (productive) cough, 5-6 leaves may be chewed from time to time, along with 2 or 3 black pepper seeds. This also clears the voice.

Enternal :-
1. A paste of the leaves when applied on the skin is effective against ringworms.
2. The same may be applied in skin diseases where itching and oozing are present.
3. The dried powder is used as a snuff in stuffy nose.
4. The paste of the entire plant may be applied over swellings to relieve pain and discomfort.
5. A paste made out of tender leaves of *tulsi* if applied over the face as a mask regularly, clears the black spots, rashes and pimples and brings life to dull skin.

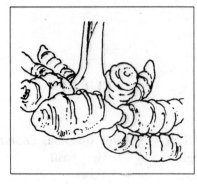

SONTH

4. SONTH — *Zingiber officinale, Zingiberaceae.*

English   -   Dried Ginger
Hindi   -   Sonth

Chief Actions :-

Stimulant of blood circulation   Promotes perspiration, menstruation
Relieves aches (as a counter-irritant)   Appetiser
Carminative

Applications :-

Internal :-

1. In loss of appetite, a decoction made by adding 1½ tsp of dry powder to a cup of water that has been boiled for 5-10 minutes, be drunk thrice a day.
2. In dyspepsia and tastelessness, a small piece of *sonth* should be eaten just before meals.
3. The same may be used in flatulence and colic pain.
4. In sore throats and hoarseness of voice, an infusion of 1 tsf of fresh root and 1 cup of boiling water may be used as a gargle.
5. In painful and swollen joints, 5 gm of dry ginger powder mixed with castor oil may be taken twice a day.

External :-

1. A warm paste may be applied over swollen and painful joints.
2. In chills and muscle cramps, dry powder and oil may be mixed and applied all over the body.
3. Rubbing dry powder over the area in oedem is very helpful.
4. In headaches, a paste is applied to the forehead for relief.

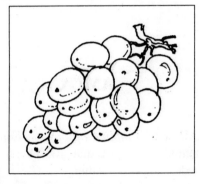

DRAKSHA

5. DRAKSHA — *Vitis vinifera, Vitaceae*
English   -   Grape/raisin
Hindi   -   Angoor

Chief Actions :-
Laxative
Coolant
Demulcent (soothing to skin and mucous membrane)

Applications :-
Internal :-
1. In burning urination, 8-10 raisins soaked in water overnight and then crushed, may be taken with sugar.
2. In thirst occurring in fevers, a few raisins boiled in water & then cooled may be taken to quench thirst and to lower the temperature.
3. In bleeding disorders, a concentrated decoction of raisins may be taken with honey and *ghee* to supplement loss of blood and to purify blood.
4. In mental disorders like intoxication and epilepsy, prolonged daily use of raisins is very effective.
5. A confection prepared with grapes, sugar, *ghee* and honey is a good tissue-vitalizer and weight-promoter.
6. It is used as a mild laxative during pregnancy.

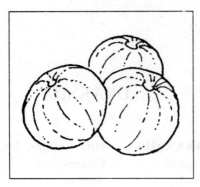

AMLA

6. AMLA — *Emblica officinalis, Euphorbiaceae*
English   -   Indian gooseberry
Hindi   -   Amla

Chief Actions :-

Cooling   Refrigerant
Diuretic   Laxative
Natural source of vitamin C   Enhances immunity

Applications :-

Internal :-

1. In burning urination, the juice taken in a dose of 10-15 ml twice a day with honey is beneficial.
2. In diarrhoea, dysentery & bleeding conditions, the dried fruits are taken, 5-10gm in dosage, twice a day with honey.
3. The same may be taken in anaemia, jaundice and indigestion owing to its high iron content.
4. It is useful in diabetes when taken as a decoction of 15ml, every morning with half-a-tsf of turmeric powder.
5. A confection prepared from the preserved fruit is useful in habitual constipation and acts as an enhancer of immunity.
   [*Chyavanprash* is a popular product consisting chiefly of *Amla*]

Enternal :-

1. A decoction of the leaves and bark is useful in mouth and tongue ulcers as a gargle.
2. Oil obtained from the berries strengthens hair and promotes hair growth.
3. In balding and greying of hair, hair is washed with the fresh juice of gooseberries.

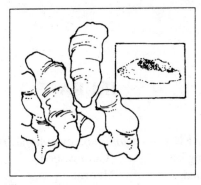

CHANDAN

7. CHANDAN — *Santalum album, Santalaceae*
English   -   Sandalwood
Hindi   -   Chandan

NOTE :- Red Sandal *(Pterocarpus santalinus* or *rakta chandan)* is used for decoctions and external applications.

Chief Actions :-
Cooling
Diuretic
Relaxant.

Applications :-
Internal :-
1. In thirst fever, decoction of sandal may be consumed from time to time to lower the temperature and to quench thirst.
2. In burning urination and bleeding of any sort, infusion of the bark powder is seen to be beneficial.
3. In skin disorders and body aches, a decoction of 15-20 ml may be taken twice a day for relief.
4. Especially in bleeding piles, 10 gm of sandal paste with 10 gm of dry ginger powder is highly beneficial.

External :-
1. A paste of the bark is applied over swellings and fresh wounds for relief from pain and burning sensation.
2. In all skin disorders, application of sandal paste reduces oozing, if any and relieves irritation and itching.
3. In prickly heat, the same may be applied for impressive results.
4. Inhaling the fragrant fumes & oil is a proven relaxant and hypotensive.
5. Used as a facepack, it improves complexion and lightens blemishes and scars.

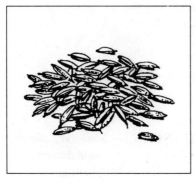

JEERA

8. JEERA — *Cuminum cyminum, Umbelliferae*
English   -   Cumin seed
Hindi   -   Jeera.

Chief Actions :-
Aromatic
Carminative
Astringent

Applications :-
Internal :-
1. White cumin seeds are given after childbirth to increase milk secretion, 10-30 grains in dosage, with jaggery.
2. In urinary calculi, dysuria and other urinary disorders, cumin powder is given with sugar.
3. In digestive disorders like intestinal colic, loss of appetite, vomiting, indigestion, flatulence and also in intestinal worm infestations, fried and powdered seeds are taken with honey, 5 gms twice a day.
4. The same powder may be taken in excessive (vaginal) white discharge, and to increase lactation in breastfeeding mothers, with milk or *ghee*.
5. In chronic fevers, powdered cumin seeds, 5gms in dosage with lukewarm water, taken twice a day for 10 days is very effective.

External :-
1. Paste of cumin seeds is highly beneficial when applied on swellings, pile masses, skin disorders and painful areas.
2. The paste, when applied on the face improves the complexion.
3. Washing the face with *jeera*-boiled-water improves the complexion and the same water may be used to wash wounds.
4. In itching and allergic rashes, this water is poured over the affected parts.

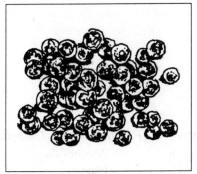

KALI MIRCH

9. KALI MIRCH — *Piper nigrum, Piperaceae*
English   -   Black Pepper
Hindi   -   Kali Mirch

Chief Actions :-
    Carminative
    Stimulant
    Counter-irritant

Applications :-

Internal :-

1. In all digestive disorders, and intestinal infections, the powder may be consumed for timely relief, 5 gm with a cup of buttermilk.
2. A decoction of pepper may be taken in cough, common cold and dyspnoea (breathing difficulty).
3. In all skin disorders with oozing and itching, the decoction is found to be useful.
4. In fever with chills, taking water boiled with pepper seeds reduces rigors and helps in lowering temperature.
5. In nervous disorders, the decoction of pepper may be taken as an effective remedy.

External :-

1. In most oozing and itching skin conditions, the paste may be applied directly or mixed with oil.
2. In conditions of pain & swelling, relief may be obtained by applying paste of pepper over the area.
3. In dental caries and toothaches, the decoction may be used as a gargle, or massaged onto the teeth and gums, or the pepper may be directly chewed.
4. In allergic rashes, pepper powder + *ghee* may be applied for relief.

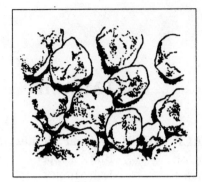

HING

10. HING — *Ferula foetida, Umbelliferae*

English	-	Asafoetida
Hindi	-	Hing

Chief Actions :-

Moderate stimulant   Anti-spasmodic

Expectorant   Vermifuge

Disinfectant

Applications :-

Internal :-

1. Raw asafoetida is given in lung infections like bronchitis, 5 gm in dosage, twice a day.
2. It is given fried in *ghee*, in all digestive disorders—loss of appetite, flatulence, colic and spasmodic pain.
3. The same is given in neuro-muscular disorders such as sciatica, facial palsy, paralysis etc., for relief from pain.
4. In urinary retention and pain in the bladder region, intake of 5gms of asafoetida fried in *ghee*, promotes normal voiding of urine.
5. In dysmenorrhoea, it may be used to promote & regulate menstruation.
6. In breathing disorders, cough and cold, it is consumed for great relief in dosages of 12-15 gm.

External :-

1. In flatulence and any digestive disorders, applying a paste of asafoetida over the abdomen gives great relief.
2. In intestinal worms, 2gm of asafoetida in 100ml of water may be used as an enema.

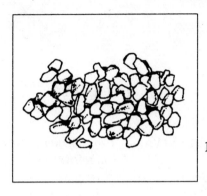

METHI

11. METHI — *Trigonella foenum graecum,*
Umbelliferae

English   -   Fenugreek
Hindi   -   Methi

Chief Actions :-

Carminative
Promotes hair growth
Relieves colic pain

Applications :-

Internal :-

1. In loss of appetite, colic, diarrhoea, dyspepsia, dysentery, the seeds may be powdered and taken.
2. To increase flow of milk in nursing mothers, the seeds may be given in the form of a gruel (*kanji*).
3. To relieve body aches, the seeds are crushed and taken.
4. The decoction of seeds may be taken in nervous debility and disorders.

External :-

1. In pain, swelling and abscesses, a paste of the seeds is warmed and applied for relief.
2. To promote hair growth, the paste of the seeds is mixed in yoghurt and applied onto the scalp.
3. The paste may be applied on burns for relief.

Caution :- It is best avoided in bleeding disorders.

141

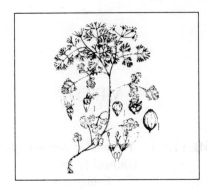

DHANIYA

12. DHANIYA — *Coriandrum sativum,*
Umbelliferae
English - Coriander
Hindi - Dhaniya

Chief Actions :-

Aromatic   Stimulant
Carminative   Antispasmodic

Applications :-
Internal :-

1. In fainting, loss of memory etc., dehusked seeds of coriander are boiled with 4 times milk and 8 times water. This is reduced to half and given twice a day.
2. In thirst, water boiled in coriander and cooled quenches thirst immediately. This is useful in diarrhoea, intestinal colic, piles and intestinal worms.
3. In cough and dyspnoea (difficulty in breathing) the decoction of the seeds may be consumed.
4. The same is beneficial in urinary problems like dysuria etc.
5. In fever accompanied by chills, it is found useful. In fever accompanied by burning sensation, thirst, etc., a cold infusion of the seeds along with sugar may be given.
6. The seeds are chewed to correct foul breath.

External :-

1. In headaches and swellings, the leaves of coriander may be applied.
2. In mouth ulcers and in throat diseases, the juice of coriander may be held in the mouth for relief.
3. In bleeding from the nose, 1-2 drops of this juice may be dropped in the nose.
4. The decoction is used to wash the eye in conjunctivitis.

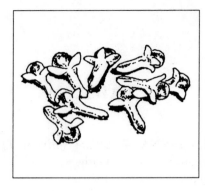

LAVANGA

13. LAVANGA — *Syzygium aromaticum,*
Myrtaceae

English   -   Clove
Hindi   -   Lavanga

Chief Actions :-

Carminative
Stimulant
Antispasmodic (relieves griping and colic pain)

Applications :-

Internal :-

In hyperacidity, vomiting, colic pain, flatulence, thirst, cough, breathing disorders and hiccups, in burning or painful urination, and to promote and clear breastmilk secretion, water boiled in cloves is regarded ideal. In all types of fevers too, the same decoction is used.

External :-

1. In headaches and colds, the paste of cloves is applied on the forehead.
2. The oil of cloves is applied to relieve sciatica, rheumatoid arthritis, and any painful joints or muscles.
3. In dental caries and toothaches, the oil is applied dipped in cotton to the teeth and gums.

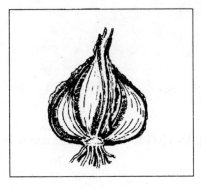

LAHSUNA

14. LAHSUNA — *Allium sativum, Liliaceae*

English	-	Garlic
Hindi	-	Lahsun

Chief Actions :-

Stimulant	Tonic
Carminative	Relieves paralysis
Gout	Sciatica

Applications :-

Internal :-

1. The aromatic oil from the seeds may be taken to prevent recurrence of cold and fever.
2. The cloves of garlic act with great benefit upon hysteria, nervous disorders and flatulence, when boiled with milk.
3. In the form of a confection in cold seasons, it eradicates rheumatism and pain in paralysis.
4. It is used to relieve from pain in arthritis and in intestinal worms and piles.
5. In dysmenorrhoea, it may be used to regulate menstruation.
6. It is beneficial in fevers of diphtheria & malaria.

External :-

1. Cloves of garlic boiled in ½ ounce of gingelly oil is useful as ear drops in earaches and atonic deafness.
2. Paste of garlic is applied in cases of facial palsy, parlaysis, body aches, swellings with pain.
3. In skin disorders with itching and oozing, rubbing with garlic paste is useful.
4. It is one of the most effective antimicrobial acting on viral, bacterial and helmentic infestations.
5. It reduces blood pressure and blood cholesterol.

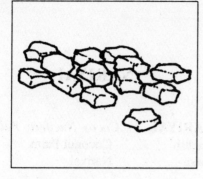

KARPOORA

15. KARPOORA — *Cinnamomum Camphora, Lauraceae*

English	-	Camphor
Hindi	-	Karpoor

Chief Actions :-

Digestive

Circulatory stimulant

Antiseptic

Relieves flatulence

Promotes perspiration

Nervous

Diuretic

Antipyretic (reduces fever)

Nervous disorders

Applications :-

Internal :-

1. In asthma, diarrhoea, coryza, cough and cold, camphor with asafoetida may be rolled into pills and consumed two pills twice a day.
2. As a prophylactic against fevers and infections, a piece may be held in the mouth everyday.
3. In uterine pains, camphor may be rolled into pills and consumed one pill thrice a day and the liniment rubbed on the abdomen.
4. An infusion of camphor may be taken in dysuria.

External :-

1. Sniffed up the nostrils, it relieves cold in the head, and the vapour inhaled through a tube, relieves chest afflictions.
2. In delirium and apoplexy, fomentation with hot water with the liniment of camphor applied to the feet and calves is beneficial.
3. In wounds, swellings, joint pains and pneumonia, the oil is used.
4. In burning feet and hands and on burns, the sprinkled powder acts as a soothing agent.
5. In degeneration of teeth and toothaches, the oil applied is relieving.
6. In chronic colds, a few drops of the volatile liquid may be dropped in the nostrils.

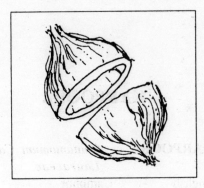

NARIYAL

16. NARIYAL — *Cocos Nucifera Palmae*

English   -   Coconut Palm

Hindi   -   Nariyal

Chief Actions :-

Nutritious

Milk of tender fruit is refrigerant

Allays gastric irritation

Applications :-

Internal :-

1. In bleeding of any sort, the water of tender coconut is beneficial, as a drink.
2. It is an excellent diuretic and promotes complexion.
3. In excessive urination and in dysentery, the flower of coconut may be consumed.
4. In dysmenorrhoea, tender coconut water as a drink provides relief from discomfort and pain.
5. In hyperacidity, the tender fruit pulp has a soothing effect on the gastric membrane.
6. The same relieves constipation and intestinal colic.

External :-

1. To lighten scars and allay burning sensation in chicken pox and measles, the lesions are washed with tender coconut water.
2. The oil from burnt kernel (outer husk of fruit) is useful in leprosy and other skin ailments.
3. The oil of fruit is an excellent promoter of hair growth and rejuvenator.
4. The same oil is also used to relieve burning sensation and dryness of skin.

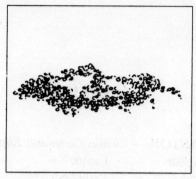

KHASKHAS

17. KHASKHAS — Seeds of *Papaver Somniferum*

English - Poppy seeds
Hindi - Posthdana/Khaskhas

Chief Actions :-

Demulcent   Nutritive
Astringent   Sedative
Narcotic

Applications :-

Internal :-

1. In all painful conditions, like sciatica, abdominal pain or colic, the seed powder with *ghee* in doses of 3gm — 2-3 times a day is beneficial.
2. In diarrhoea, the paste of the seeds ground in water, 3gm — 2-3 times a day is useful.
3. In loss of sleep, the same may be taken for good results.
4. In all nervous disorders, the decoction of the seeds, 20-25 ml twice a day is beneficial.
5. In cough and asthma, the seeds may be consumed for great benefit.

External :-

1. In joint pains, pleuritis and all swellings and painful conditions, the paste is applied for relief or fomentation or poultice is made of the seeds and applied.
2. In inflammatory conditions of the eye or ear, a paste of the seeds may be applied around the eyes or ears for great relief.
3. In cold rigors or chills, the paste is applied locally.

Caution :- This may be best avoided in pregnant and breast feeding women and in children. Also avoid in large doses and for long durations.

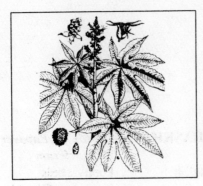

CASTOR

18. CASTOR — *Ricinus Communis Euphorbiaceae*

English   -   Castor

Hindi   -   Redi/Andi

Chief Actions :-

Purgative

Arrests bleeding

Applications :-

Internal :-

1. The oil is given in most nervous disorders like sciatica, paralysis, neuritis, facial palsy & joint pains. *Dose* : 5 ml twice a day.
2. The same is useful in digestive disorders as a purgative and corrective. It is quite beneficial in conditions of intestinal worms and hernia.
3. In pain in the bladder region and urinary disorders, the oil acts as a soothing and corrective agent.
4. Diluted 3 times with a bland oil, it is useful in rheumatic pains. *Dose* : 5 ml twice a day.
5. In swellings and body aches, internal use of the oil gives good results.

External :-

1. A paste made of the leaves of wild castor is applied on the breast to increase breastmilk secretion.
2. The fresh juice of the stem is applied to arrest bleeding from wounds, ulcers, cuts etc.
3. The stems of the plant act as toothbrushes and are used to strengthen gums and to cure spongy gums and gum boils.
4. In skin diseases, nervous disorders and swellings, external application with the oil is highly recommended, or the leaves warmed and tied with a cloth on the affected parts.

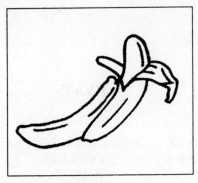

KELA

19. KELA — *Musa Sapientum, Scitaminae*
English - Banana
Hindi - Kela

Chief Actions :-
Coolant
Laxative
Acts against scurvy

Applications :-
Internal :-
1. As a diet in bleeding disorders.
2. As a laxative, in constipation, bananas taken on empty stomach early in the morning ensure free passage of stools.
3. In dried state, the fruit combats scurvy.
4. In hyperacidity, heartburn and colic, the ash of the leaves and stalks, 5gm twice or thrice a day is a great reliever.
5. The root powder is given in anaemic conditions. *Dose* : 5gm twice a day.
6. In bleeding from rectum/genitals, the juice of the tender roots may be taken, 20ml in dosage, twice a day.
7. When mixed with ghee and sugar, the fruit pulp relieves urinary retention.
8. In dysmenorrhoea and menorrhaegia the juice of the flowers with yoghurt is highly beneficial.

External :-
1. The tender leaves with oil may be applied to soothe blistered and inflamed skin.
2. The fruit pulp acts as a good face mask.
3. The juice of the root with borax may be used to wash wounds and ulcers.

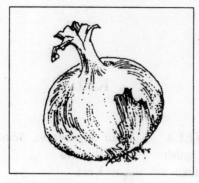

PYAZ

20. PYAZ — *Allium Cepa, Liliaceae*

English   -   Onion bulb
Hindi   -   Pyaz

Chief Actions :-

Stimulant   Diuretic
Expectorant   Rubefacient

Applications :-

Internal :-

1. In malarial fevers, 10-15gm of onion pulp along with a few black peppers twice a day is recommended.
2. In jaundice, spleen enlargement and indigestion, the same may be taken, preserved or cooked in vinegar.
3. An onion bulb fried in *ghee* and sprinkled with a little sugar may be taken in piles with great benefit.
4. The fresh juice is taken in fever and dropsy in doses of 20ml twice a day.
5. In scurvy, the same may be taken with a little salt.
6. It is very effective as an expectorant in cough.
7. As a prophylactic against sunstroke, plaque and infectious diseases, chewing onions is quite beneficial.
8. The juice also acts as a diuretic.

External :-

1. The juice may be used as a smelling salt in fainting, hysteria and fits.
2. As eardrops in earaches, the juice is effective.
3. Mixed with mustard oil, onion juice is a good application for rheumatic pains.
4. Onion bulbs are roasted and applied as a poultice on boils and swellings.
5. Smelling the onion bulb is in itself protective against sunstroke.
6. The juice is warmed and applied on patches on the skin.
7. It is used to relieve itching and oozing in skin diseases.

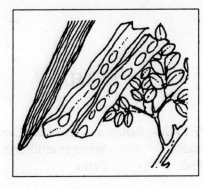

DRUMSTICK

21. DRUMSTICK — *Moringa Oleifera,*
Moringaceae

English - Horse radish tree/Drumstick tree
Hindi - Sahijan/Munga

Chief Actions :-

Emmenogogue   Digestive
Carminative   Reduces colic

Applications :-

Internal :-

1. In loss of appetite, colic pain and flatulence, the seeds may be used for great benefit.
2. In dysmenorrhoea or in scanty menstruation, the decoction of the seeds or leaves may be used.
3. In burning sensation while passing urine, the decoction of the seeds may be used.
4. A hot infusion of the leaves may be consumed in skin diseases for great relief.
5. In fever with chills, the same is indicated to reduce temperature.

External :-

1. The paste of the root is given in swellings and abscesses.
2. In headaches, the powder of the seeds is dropped in the nostrils.
3. The oil of the seeds is used to reduce pains & swelling and as an application in arthritic and rheumatic pains.

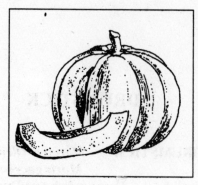

PETHA

22. PETHA—*Benincasa Hispida, Cucurbitaceae.*
English - White gourd/Pumpkin
Hindi - Petha

Chief Actions :-
Brain tonic
Coolant
Nutritive

Applications :-
Internal :-
1. It is an excellent brain tonic—enhances memory and is useful in all psychological and psychiatric disorders.
2. In chronic thirst and intestinal worms, the seed oil is used in a dose of 10-20 ml with great benefit.
3. In bleeding piles and bleeding disorders the fresh juice may be taken from time to time.
4. The ash of the seeds is useful in colicky pain. *Dose:* ½ tsp twice a day with *ghee.*
5. In constipation, a confection of the flesh of the fruit may be taken habitually.
6. As a coolant drink, the juice beats the heat in summer and relieves thirst and urinary retention.
7. In chronic fever, it relieves burning sensation and reduces body temperature.

External :-
1. In burns, the flesh of the fruit is applied locally. The juice of the leaves may be used to relieve burning sensation.
2. The seed oil is used as a coolant in headache associated with burning sensation.

152

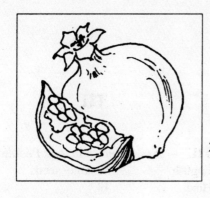

ANAR

23. ANAR — *Punica Granatum, Punicaceae*
English   -   Pomegranate
Hindi   -   Anar

Chief Actions :-
Anthelmentic
Astringent

Applications :-
Internal :-
1. In hyperacidity, diarrhoea, & low appetite, it is of great benefit to take the peel off the fruit, dried and powdered in doses of 5-10gm, twice or thrice a day.
2. In children's diarrhoea, the buds are to be given with goat's milk.
3. In worms, especially tapeworm infestations, the decoction of the root— 10-20gm in dosage is taken, followed by a purgative.
4. In all the blood disorders, the fresh juice of the fruit along with the peel acts as a blood purifier.
5. In dry cough, the fruits may be taken.
6. The fresh fruit juice is also given in urinary disorders.
7. It is useful as a diet in fevers.

External :-
1. To wash wounds and ulcers, the juice is highly useful.
2. A gargle of the decoction of the fruit peel is highly beneficial in throat and oral afflictions.

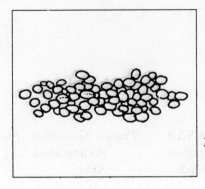

TIL

24. TIL — *Sesamum Indicum, Pedaliaceae*

English - Sesame seeds

Hindi - Til

Chief Actions :-
Emollient

Demulcent

Laxative

Applications :-
Internal :-

1. In the form of a decoction or sweetmeat, it is quite useful in constipation.
2. In cases of amenorrhoea and dysmenorrhoea, the powdered seeds are to be taken in doses of 5gm 3 times a day along with a warm hip bath containing a handful of the bruised seeds.

External :-

1. In loosening of teeth and speech defects, gargling with *til* oil has to be done for a few days.
2. The oil is used for dressing wounds.
3. The oil forms a good base for many medicated body and hair oils since it promotes hair growth and blackens the hair.
4. In cracked feet, it should be applied daily after duly cleaning the affected feet.

Caution :- This should be avoided during pregnancy.

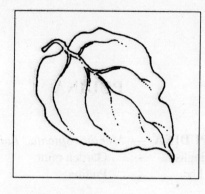

PAN LEAVES

25. PAN LEAVES — *Piper Betal, Piperaceae*

English - Beetel leaves
Hindi - Pan ke Patte

Chief Actions :-

Carminative   Aromatic
Astringent   Expectorant
Relieves stomach ache   Fever

Applications :-

Internal :-

1. Chewing of the leaves is effective against catarrhal afflictions, inflammation of the throat & bronchitis.
2. 10-15 ml of juice of the leaves mixed with milk is given in hysteria.
3. The tender leaves with black pepper are used in productive cough.

External :-

1. The juice of the leaves is dropped in the ear to relieve earaches.
2. Leaves smeared with oil, warmed and applied over the chest in bronchitis is beneficial.

155

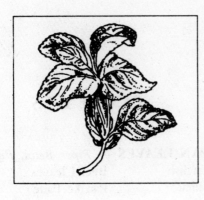

PUDINA

26. PUDINA — *Mentha Spicata, Labiatae*
English   -   Garden mint
Hindi   -   Pudina

Chief Actions :-

Aromatic   Carminative
Antispasmodic   Stimulant

Applications :-

Internal :-
1. An infusion of the leaves is used in doses of 1-2 tsf thrice a day in conditions of indigestion, loss of appetite or tastelessness.
2. The same decoction is useful as an emmenogogue (to stimulate menstruation) in dysmenorrhoea.
3. The juice of the leaves is useful for relief from hyperacidity.

External :-
1. The juice is used on ulcerated skin to heal it.

Caution :- Large doses are avoided during pregnancy.

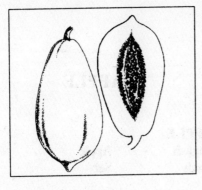

PAPAYA

27. PAPAYA — *Carica Papaya Caricaceae*
English - Papaya
Hindi - Papita

Chief Actions :-

Green fruit acts as laxative
Diuretic
Emmenogogue
Anthelmentic

Applications :-

Internal :-
1. Ripe fruit when eaten regularly corrects habitual constipation.
2. Ripe fruit regulates menstrual periods in women.
3. The unripe fruit is useful in promoting lactation in breastfeeding mothers.
4. The fruit in combination with some salt is taken twice a day when suffering from enlarged spleen and liver.
5. An infusion of the leaves is given in doses of 20ml twice a day, in dysuria.

External :-
1. The fresh milky juice acts as a promoter of blood circulation and is also useful in ringworm and other skin infections.
2. The heated leaves are applied on painful areas to relieve pain.

Caution :- Unripe fruit and sap are to be avoided by pregnant women and in bleeding.

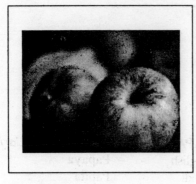

APPLE

28. APPLE

English	-	Apple
Hindi	-	Seb

Applications :-

Internal :-

1. Apple juice together with honey and milk is very useful in nervous debility.
2. Apple juice with honey is effective in pregnancy anaemia.
3. Apple, due to its property of stimulating saliva is advisable to patients of ulcer.
4. Apple is good in tooth infections and in diarrhoea and dysentery.
5. Apple along with banana regulates bowel movements.
6. Eating an apple after a non-vegetarian diet helps in easy digestion.

External :-

1. A paste made from apple leaves, used as a shampoo prevents hairfall and dandruff and promotes hair growth.
2. Application of the pulp of apple on the eyelids for an hour reduces the strain on eyes caused by overreading or sun radiation.
3. Apple pulp applied on the face cures acne and improves the complexion.

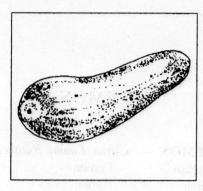

CUCUMBER

29. CUCUMBER — *Cucumis Sativus-*
Cucurbitaceae

English - Cucumber
Hindi - Kheera

Chief Actions :-
Demulcent
Coolant
Mild diuretic
Seeds—anthelmentic

Applications :-
Internal :-
1. The leaves in a dose of 15gm act as a diuretic.
2. The fruit is cooling and healing on ulcers of the gastrointestinal tract.
3. The oil obtained from the seeds acts as a tonic and diuretic.
4. The powdered seeds given in a dose of 3-5gm is useful as a vitalizer in general debility.

External :-
1. Cucumber gel is popularly used as a facepack to smoothen skin and improve general complexion.
2. In summer, the slices of cucumber placed over eyes help relax and freshen them.
3. The juice of the fruit is useful in burning sensation of the skin.

159

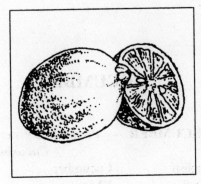

LEMON

30. LEMON — *Citrus Limon Rutaceae*

English	-	Lemon
Hindi	-	Nimbu

Chief Actions :-
Refrigerant
bleaching agent

Applications :-

Internal :-

1. The fruit acts as a refrigerant and is therefore useful in conditions of burning sensation.
2. The juice is taken 10ml in quantity, in conditions of ulcers of mouth, spongy gums, pyorrhoea and other oral problems.
3. Lemon juice along with honey is used daily early in the morning, to clear abdominal discomfort and as a blood purifier.
4. The same preparation also helps reduce weight.

External :-

1. Lemon juice along with yoghurt is an effective topical application against dandruff.
2. The powder of lemon peel is used as a facepack in oily skin condition.
3. Lemon juice is a good bleaching agent, and is therefore widely used as an ingredient in facepacks.

Part-III
Nature Cure at Home

1. MEDICATED MASSAGES

For centuries oil massage has been part of the routine of Indian households. A 'keep-fit' tradition enjoyed by everyone from babies to great grandmothers, it is an excellent way to combat the stress of modern life.

How does massage keep you fit and healthy? It is explained hereunder:
* Increases circulation and provides body tissues with more oxygen.
* Relaxes muscles and helps ease stress and tension.
* Eases stiffness in joints.
* Tones the body keeping it supple and young.
* Helps flush out wastes from the body.
* Stimulates and tones the skin.
* Increases energy and vitality.
* Makes you feel good!

The oil massage is a great way to start each day. It should not be rushed; so try and give yourself some time to do it leisurely, and follow it with a warm bath. Since mornings tend to be hectic, you might prefer to do it in the evening when you have more time for yourself.

THE TRADITIONAL HEAD-TO-TOE SELF-MASSAGE ROUTINE

Start with the head and work your way down, using upward strokes at the back of the body and downward strokes at the front. Circular motions should be clockwise. This is said to release tension. Use natural oils.

THE HEAD

The face: Oil fingertips and massage from centre of the face, outwards and put some oil on the centre of your head and massage into the scalp towards ears with fingertips of both hands? Keep fingers behind the first spot, put some more oil and repeat the procedure. Next bend the head forward and put some oil where the back of the head meets the neck and rub towards the ears. Gently tap the whole head with your fists. Then rub the entire scalp gently pulling at your hair upwards starting from the forehead. Finish below the jaw, gently kneading the jawline.
The neck: Keep hands well oiled for massaging the rest of the body. With the right hand stroke up the left side of the back of the neck. Do the same with the left hand for the right side simultaneously. Stroke down the front with both hands. Avoid pressing the wind pipe.
The arms: With the right hand, massage shoulder, elbow and wrist of left arm with small circular motions. Work down the inside of the arm, along muscle curves. Continue up the back of the arm, up towards shoulders. Repeat same procedure on the other arm.

163

The hands: Stroke down the back of the hands, pulling each finger. With thumb, massage palms working up to the base of the fingers.

The body: With the palm of the hands, starting from the shoulder, massage the front with large circular movements upwards and outwards. Massage abdomen in clockwise circles starting from belly button. Massage the back from the base of the spine working upwards and outwards from the spine. Finish by squeezing the top of the shoulders. Massage the buttocks in large clockwise circles.

The legs: Apply oil generously to the legs. Use both hands to massage each leg, one hand on the inside and one on the outside. Starting from the hip, stroke down the front upper leg. Stroke upwards from just above the knee on the back of the leg. Stroke down the front of the lower leg from knee to ankle and then up the back of the leg from ankle to knee.

The feet: Stroke down the foot and pull each toe (similar to hand massage). Massage the soles and heels generously with oil and rub well. Finish with a gentle circular rub at the centre of your feet. Follow your massage with a small rest and then a warm bath.

OTHER FORMS OF MASSAGE

1. Swedish Massage: Though based on oriental techniques, Swedish massage is the first system of therapeutic massage in the Western world; developed around the eighteenth century. It primarily aims at speeding up venous return of deoxygenated and toxic blood from the extremities. Some specific strokes have been incorporated for this purpose. Swedish massage improves blood circulation, stretches the ligaments and tendons while also relaxing the nervous system.

2. Reichian Massage: It was developed by a psychologist William Reich, who believed that the body stores past emotions and psychological traumas in localized areas, blocking the vital life force energy. By massaging these blocked areas, this blocked vital force is psychologically released.

3. Acupressure Massage: Also known as "Shiatsu" or finger pressure massage, it is based on the Chinese theory of "Chi", the subtle energy circulating in the body meridians. This energy may be manipulated on specific points along the meridians, by varying pressure, stretching and rubbing. It deals with a level of body energy higher than just gross physical joints and muscles.

All these procedures though, may be performed only by experts.

2. SPECIAL FOMENTATION METHODS

These procedures include hydrotherapy, hot water bottle compresses, ice bags etc. The skin is the main site of application. By thermally, mechanically and chemically stimulating the skin, various reflexes may be activated.

These may be applied both on sick and healthy individuals.

HOT Body Temperature	COLD Body Temperature
Though the entire body responds to heat the response is more at the site of application.	Though the entire body responds to cold, the response is more at the site of application.
Effects: Applied to the skin, draws blood from the internal organs. (Applied to the heart region, it increases pulse rate)	**Effects:** Applied to the skin, it sends blood flow to the internal organs. (Applied to the heart region, pulse rate decreases, and pain in the heart is relieved)
Perspiration caused by heat also results in the breakdown of exudate in inflammations.	Application of cold retards development of acute inflammations.

HYDROTHERAPY

Showers, baths, sponging, wet packs and similar procedures can be done at home with great benefits.

1. **Pouring:** To fortify the patient's body, water can be poured over the body from a pail. For overall fortification, the patient is seated on a low stool in a bath tub or room and water which is tolerably hot (to the patient) is first poured in continuous streams and then the temperature of the water is gradually lowered to lukewarm. The body should be rubbed dry until it reddens slightly. This procedure can be done as a prelude to an oil massage or any face/body pack.

2. **Water Sprayed with a Hose:** This procedure is applied usually only to the back and the legs. The jet of water is sprayed along the backbone for about 5 minutes to improve the general tone.

3. **Rubbing:** This is yet another hydrotherapeutic procedure which can be used during fever neurosis. This can be general or local.

    a) For a general procedure, a bedsheet wetted in hot water is wrapped around the patient's naked body — first layer under his arms and the next over his shoulders and finally fixed to the neck. The patient's body is rubbed vigorously through the sheet for 2-3 minutes, after which the wet sheet is replaced by a dry one.

b) For weak patients the same is done locally on body parts. This procedure improves general circulation and can also be done before an oil massage and in conditions of numbness, dryness and chills.

4. **Packs:** They can be wet or dry, local or general.
   General: a) A wet sheet (soaked in hot water) is placed on a cot already covered with a couple of blankets. The patient is undressed and placed on this sheet, wrapped — similar to the above procedure. The patient is retained in this position for an hour to two.

   This procedure is effective against early hypertension and neurosis.

   Local: b) Local Packs are used for obesity, i.e. the patient is wrapped to the waist. Dry packs are effective in such cases.

5. **Baths:** They are general or local. Depending on the temperature of water, baths may be cold, lukewarm or hot. They may be plain/medicated.

   Hot baths intensify metabolism and sweating. They also relax the muscles and remove pain.

   They are highly useful in renal, intestinal and other colic pains.

   Contra Indications: Heart diseases, bleeding disorders and asthenia of skin, joints and muscles.

6. **Showers:** This continuous spray of water (in several jets) can be had from an overhead hand shower, and acts through two factors — thermal and mechanical.

   a) Short cold showers increase muscle and vascular tone.
   b) Prolonged hot and cold showers decrease excitability of the nervous system and speed up metabolism.
   c) Warm showers produce a quieting effect. An energetic scrubbing is indicated after showering to intensify blood circulation in the skin.

FOMENTATION METHODS

Fomentation is a simple, easy to follow method both for the healthy and for those seeking quick relief from minor ailments. Based on different ways of applying heat, Ayurveda divides fomentation/sudation (process of inducing sweat) into 4 categories.

1. **Direct Heat:** This is a method of applying heat to the affected parts by means of heated cloth bundles, in which either sand, salt or medicinal leaves (like castor, *madar*, neem, lemon, *sambhalu*) are tied. Oil is first smeared on the site, and the bundles, heated intermittently on a hot pan to tolerable temperature are applied (so as not to scald the skin) for 15-20 minutes. This is done everyday for about a week to 15 days.

Note:
1. Sand works best in rheumatoid arthritis.
2. Salt provides great relief in conditions of pain and stiffness.

3. In cases of cold, cough and breathing difficulty in children, heat produced by rubbing both palms together should be applied on the chest, throat and back for about 10 minutes.

Even hot water bags fall under this category which is called *Tapa* in Ayurvedic parlance.

2. **Warm Poultices and Compresses:** A compress can be made by squeezing out a ball of cotton wool in hot water or in a decoction of castor leaves, and applying on the affected joints for 15-20 minutes.

A poultice acts just like a compress — only it remains hot for a longer time. It can be made by packing overcooked rice (thick *kanji*) and the above mentioned herbs with salt and oil in 2 layers of cloth and then bandaging the cloth on the affected area with a piece of warm cloth or leather. A single poultice can be left on for a maximum of 6-8 hours after which a fresh one should be applied. This is known as Upanaha as per Ayurveda.

3. **Steaming:** It is best for relief from sinusitis, bronchitis, common cold, wet cough and attacks of bronchial asthma.

Water boiled in eucalyptus, *tulsi, karpura* and belladonna may be used for the purpose. Steaming should be done for a maximum of 15-20 minutes.

CAUTION: The eyes should always be protected by a piece of cloth during steaming.

This is called *Ushma* according to Ayurveda.

4. **Hot Water Baths:** [See Hydrotherapy] Commonly known as a tub bath, this procedure yields good results in piles, dysuria, painful diseases and other diseases affecting the area below the navel. This is called *Drava* as per Ayurveda.

CAUTION: All the above procedures should be avoided in conditions of burning sensation, bleeding, fainting and in suppurating ulcers.

---

3. HINTS FOR POSITIVE HEALTH

Health or wellness, is a state of being, a feeling that is experienced. (Feeling happy is health). Ayurveda in a nutshell says *Sukha Sangnakam Aarogyan* — that is, a feeling of happiness and comfort is health.

The World Health Organisation defines Health as "state of being, that is, not merely the absence of disease, but a state of complete physical, mental and social well-being". This broad-based definition of health suggests a continuum that ranges from death to diseased states (poor health) to freedom from disease to perfect health. Our health at any point of time lies somewhere on the scale indicated below.

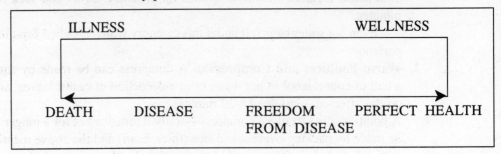

THE HEALTH CONTINUUM

Why does one need a longer and healthy span of life? What are the *objectives* of human life? Most of us immediately think of meaningful employment, money, fame, intimate and loving relationships, possessions, etc. The one element all these goals have in common is *Happiness*.

Sound Health is the 'basis' for happiness. And the following are the useful hints of Ayurveda for attainment of Perfect Health. If one follows these principles in *toto* in everyday life, one is one hundred per cent assured of good health, the fountain of Happiness.

THE DAILY REGIMEN

Ayurveda advocates a definite daily regimen to maintain health and ward off disease.

1. **Waking Up:** At *Brahma Muhurta*, that is around 4:30 A.M., since the atmosphere is clean, fresh and rich in oxygen.

2. **Brushing Teeth:** With twigs of bitter drugs like *khadira, arjuna, neem* etc.
   Avoidance: The use of a toothbrush is best avoided in persons suffering from indigestion, dyspnoea, cough, fever, facial paralysis, ulceration of mouth, and heart, ear and head diseases. Brushing is followed by gargling, inhalation of fumes of *hing, guggul, tulsi,* etc.

3. **Chewing Betel:** This is best done after meals to give a feeling of satisfaction and also to help digestion.
   Avoidance: It is contra-indicated in those suffering from wounds, bleeding diseases, redness of the eyes, poisoning, those in unconscious state or intoxication and in those suffering from constipation.

4. **Daily Massage:** Gingelly oil is considered best to be applied daily all over the body accompanied by a light massage. This wards off old age, relieves exertion, bestows glowing skin, long life and sound sleep. Application of oil should be done especially to the head, ears and feet.
   Avoidance: Still it is best avoided in conditions of indigestion, fever, cold, etc.

5. **Exercise:** Physical exercise, tolerable to the individual, when done daily, bestows ability to do work, keen digestion, melts excess fat and makes the body compact. *Avoidance*: Very small children, the very old and those suffering from burning sensation, and painful conditions should best avoid it. Exercise should be followed by a light massage of the exerted body parts.

6. **Powder Massage:** Using soft fragrant powders e.g. a mixture of sandalwood powder and *besan*, to rub on to the body is seen to liquefy fat, produces stability of body parts and bestows glowing skin.

7. **Bath:** Pouring hot water on the body bestows strength, but the same should be avoided on the head as it causes hair fall and eye-related problems (lukewarm water should be used on the head).
   Avoidance: It is best avoided immediately after food and in conditions of indigestion, facial palsy, diseases of the eyes, mouth and ears (wherein a hot water sponge can substitute a bath).

GENERAL TIPS

1. Generally, food should be taken only after the previous meal is digested, and in limited quantities.
2. The bodily urges such as urination, defecation, sneezes, cough, belching, flatulence, etc., should never be either controlled or forced out.

Apart from these hints for physical health, Ayurveda also gives tips on good conduct:

1. While speaking, it must be made sure that the words are relevant, brief, true and agreeable.
2. While beginning a conversation, the face should be pleasant, attentive and pleasing to others. While listening, one need not believe everything one has heard nor suspect every word that one has heard, that is to say, having an open mind is best. It is useful to avoid controversial topics like previous insults, personal enmities and unpleasantries between one's employee and oneself.
3. One's sense organs should not be overstrained, at the same time not overindulged either.
4. One should wear clothes that fit well, and appear well groomed, without causing the impression of being flamboyant.
5. In all matters taking the mid path and avoiding the extremes yields best results.
6. One should not sneeze, laugh or yawn without covering one's mouth.
7. One should not unnecessarily blow his nose or fidget with objects, to avoid creating a nervous impression.
8. One should stop the activities of body, speech and mind before reaching the point of exhaustion.
9. One should not gaze at the sun for a long time nor carry heavy objects on the head, nor strain the eyes staring at very small shining objects.

10. One should avoid direct onslaught of winds, sunlight, dust, snow etc.
11. One should not sneeze, belch, cough, eat or sleep in awkward postures.

These do's and don'ts, as is obvious, are quite relevant to today's lifestyle too, and help maintain the body's positive health and immunity.

Stay "Seasoned" — not "Weather-beaten" : Seasonal regimes:

To maintain bodily balance, it is necessary to make the required adjustments in food and behaviour, according to the seasonal variations. Some useful tips are given below:

1. **Winter:** Use of sweet, sour and salt tastes in food is beneficial. All sorts of procedures with medicated oils like mild massages are advised during this season, followed by bathing in warm water (boiled in *aguru*, musk and *kesar*). Rich/Fatty foods can be consumed, thick apparel should be worn and all indoor activities can be resorted to.

2. **Spring:** Light non-fatty foods and physical exercises are beneficial. Preparation for the summer by anointing the body with cold fragrant substances like sandal, camphor pasted with honey is advised. It is judicious to avoid fatty, sour and sweet tastes in food, and sleeping during daytime. (Alcohol may be consumed in moderation).

3. **Summer:** All salty, pungent and sour food should be avoided. Cool, sweet, light and liquid food is the most suitable diet in summer. Protection from the scorching heat is desirable, at all times, and clothing should be minimal, light and comfortable.

4. **Monsoon:** Since this season renders the body prone to many diseases, care should be taken to steer clear of the muddy, murky water, and to remain unexposed to the torrent of the skies. Exposing the body to warm fumes of camphor, *guggul* etc., is highly recommended.

5. **Autumn:** Lean meats, bitter and sweet foods are advised. Strong liquids, exposure to the sun and wind, and heavy meals including fries and yoghurt are best avoided.

These suggestions, when followed appropriately, definitely help combat the seasonal onslaught of diseases and restore balance to the body.

FIBRE AND HEALTH

Dietary fibre can be easily defined as anything that moves through the gastro-intestinal tract and is not digested as food.

Growing awareness on the need to put fibre back into one's diet is a result of evidence, pointing to processed and refined foods as the culprit for many a disease characteristic of urban and rich societies.

The major source of dietery fibre is plant cell wall material which is not digested by human enzymes.

On the contrary, flour and sugar, high-energy but low-fibre foods are being blamed for causing disease in two ways: 1. Altered intestinal function and 2. Increased energy intake leading to obesity and diabetes.

How the body absorbs carbohydrates:

1. Sugar, soft drinks — *shoot* into the blood.
2. Starches, bread, potatoes — *stream* into the blood.
3. Fruits - *flow* into the blood.
4. Carbohydrates made from milk — *drip* into the blood.
5. Vegetables (fibre rich) — *seep* into the blood.

Diseases that are avoided by a fibre rich diet:

1. Constipation and therefore hernia and varicose veins.
2. Carcinoma of bowel.
3. Cancer of colon.
4. Haemorrhoids/piles.
5. Diverticular disease.
6. Atherosclerosis and thereby heart attacks.

What fibre does:

1. Maintains bacterial population of intestine.
2. Speeds passage of food residues through digestive tract.
3. Increases and softens waste matter, encouraging production of vitamins.

HEALTH EATING

Do eat lots of	Do not eat too much of
Whole-grain cereals	Refined bakes and confectionaries
Fruits	Sugar
Raw vegetables	Fat meat (Lean meat, liver preferred)
Nuts and leaves	Fried foods

COMMON HIGH FIBRE FOODS

Grains Fruits	Vegetables	Pulses	Nuts and Oil seeds	
Rice bran	Drumsticks	Green gram	Coconut	Guava
Ragi	Beans	Peas gram	Sunflower seeds	Dates
Oatmeal	Peas	Bengal gram	Gingelly seeds	*Amla*
Maize	Cluster beans	Soyabean	Groundnuts	*Bael*
Barley	Cauliflower	Low pea		Grapes
Whole wheat	Tamarind			Lemon
Hand-pounded Rice	Carrot			Apple
	Curry leaves			

Spices: Cardamoms, *jeera,* pepper, nutmeg, ginger, fresh asafoetida.

4. HOMELY BEAUTY AIDS

AYURVEDA AND SKIN

Ayurveda, the Indian System of Medicine categorised our constitution otherwise called Prakriti mainly under Vata, Pitta and Kapha.

KAPHA PRAKRITI	PITTA PRAKRITI	VATA PRAKRITI
1. Thick, moist, pale	1. Fair, peachy	1. Thin, fine-pored
2. Soft and cool to touch	2. Soft, lustrous	2. Cool to touch
3. Tones well and ages gracefully	3. Chemically sensitive	3. Sensitive to touch

KAPHA VIKRITI	PITTA VIKRITI	VATA VIKRITI
1. Dull, sluggish	1. Rashes, Itching	1. Lack of tone, lustre
2. Enlarged pores	2. Oily T-Zone	2. Dry rashes
3. Thick oily secretions	3. Acne, black heads	3. Corns and calluses
	4. Pigmentation	4. Dry eczema

172

Skin care, therefore varies from person to person depending on his/her constitution. When the system is out of balance, the condition is termed *Vikriti*.

Ayurveda offers excellent regenerative therapy for the skin including massage, steaming, scrubbing (with *Ubtan*/mild abrasives).

- **MASSAGE:** Massage loosens toxins and tones the muscles. Oils like sesame, sunflower, almond and apricot are used as media along with other essential oils depending on the *Dosha* involved.
  * **VATA:** Some of the essential and beneficial materials for *Vata*: Clay, sage, geranium, jasmine, orange, rose and sandalwood.
    Carrier Oils: Carrot seed, avocado.
  * **PITTA:** Rosewood, sandalwood, jasmine and rose oils.
    Carrier Oils: Coconut oil, sunflower oil and sesame oil.
  * **KAPHA:** Cedar, musk, cinnamon.
    Carrier Oils: Mustard, olive and almond.

After oil massage, warm compresses or steaming is given with herbals like bay-leaf, licorice, fennel, lavender, lemon peel, ginger mint and orange peel with the essential oils. This is to let the oil seep into the skin and nourish it.

LISTEN TO THE LANGUAGE OF SKIN

One must learn to listen to skin language. There should be no burning, itching, irritation, redness or peeling of skin after use of any cosmetics or soaps or powders.

- **UBTAN:** A good massage is followed by *Ubtan* made of a mixture of these herbals, oat flour, powdered almonds, *tulsi* powder, rose petals, lily petals, sandalwood and coriander seeds.
- **MASK:** After the scrub, a mask is usually applied to clean, nourish and tone the skin. Clay is considered to be the best mask for all types of skin. Face packs are masks for the face.
- **FACEPACK:** A good facepack for normal and dry skin can be made with one part of mineral clay to which a little aloe juice and honey are added. Water can be added up for consistency.

The same pack can be altered a little for oily skins by adding a teaspoon of aloe juice and another of lime juice.

A good toning routine should preferably have non-alcoholic ingredients. Rose water is a very good toner for all types of skin. This can be followed by a herbal moisturiser prepared from:

2 tablespoons	Aloe vera gel
1 oz	Lanchin
2 ounces	Water
2 ounces	Jejube oil

173

Using a spray mist made from equal amounts of herbal tea and mineral water will help remove dead cells and regenerate the skin to a large extent.

- *Pressure Oint Massage*: A light pressure point massage with unsalted home made butter will help in reducing dark circles under the eyes and provide relief from eye strain.

Ayurvedic treatment is not common to everybody. Every person's living conditions, mental make up individually are carefully analysed and only then drugs are prescribed.

SAVE YOUR SKIN
- Chocolates coffee, cigarettes and high fat food are real no-nos for good skin.
- Ultraviolet Rays are most intense between 11 AM and 3 PM when the sun is at its peak. Avoid direct exposure to sunlight.

SKIN PACKS FOR GLOWING SKIN

• FOR NORMAL SKIN

Blend equal quantities of sandalwood powder, rose petal powder and oat flour with milk and dab on.

• FOR DRY SKIN

Mix equal amounts of green gram powder, wheat gram power, fenugreek, *tulsi* powder and rose petals with milk cream and apply.

• FOR OILY SKIN

Mix equal quantities of rice powder, coriander seed powder, *neem* powder and sandalwood powder with water and apply.

- Normal acids (alpha-hydroxy-acids) found in fruits, sugarcane and milk, applied to any type of skin remove dead cells and stimulate blood circulation.

SKIN

HONEY: Spread a thin layer of honey on your face to soften harsh lines on skin. Wipe out with cotton wool soaked in warm water after 20 minutes.

JEERA: Washing the face with *jeera*-boiled water improves complexion.

LEMON JUICE: A mixure of lemon juice and rose water in the proportion of 1:2 is ideal to get rid of the dull grey skin on your elbows and knees.

VINEGAR: A small cup of vinegar added in your bath water will help refresh dry skin.

MILK: Dab milk onto your face with some cottonwool. Wash off after 30 minutes for a smooth even complexion.

YOGHURT: Applying yoghurt on your face as well as arms and legs, softens the skin. It is also a great coolant, especially, when you have just come back from an outing in the sun.

* Yoghurt may be mixed with rice flour to ease out cracks in the body.

* It may be combined with *chana ata* (gram flour) to dry out pimples.
* For best results, do not refrigerate yoghurt. Use when fresh. With vinegar, it relieves cracked soles.

APPLE: Slice an apple finely and spread all over your face. Excellent toner for dry skin.

TOMATO: Apply on blackheads, open pores and greasy skin.

CABBAGE: Save the water that cabbage has been cooked in, to wash your face with. It is a rich source of vitamins and minerals.

CARROT: Boil some carrots and mash into a paste. Apply and leave this on your skin for 10-15 minutes and rinse off with milk. The vitamin A in carrots is a great nourisher.

POTATO: Save the water that potato has been boiled in to wash your face with, for its nourishment.

ALUM: A fine yellowish or whitish powder with astringent properties used mainly in cleaning. Alum may be gently rubbed on the skin, after washing to remove accumulated grime and sweat. Being a mild antiseptic, its solution in water may be used as an aftershave lotion too.

ALMONDS: Make a fine paste of almonds adding a bit of rose water and make a nourishing face mask.

OIL: May be blended with home made creams for skin care as a base.

BUTTER MILK: May be used as a cleaner and for bleaching out slight discolourations, especially good for oily skin.

CAMPHOR: A white crystalline substance, it can be used as a smoothening agent on spots and as an antiseptic.

CAMPHOR OIL: Instantly relieves aching muscles. Specially mixed in massage creams as warm up.

CLOVES: An aromatic spice used in skin preparations and face mask.

CUCUMBER: A home vegetable, it cools and refreshes, when sliced circular pieces are gently stroked over the face on sunny days. It can be blended with lotions, masks and creams.

EGG-YOLK: May be used as a nourishing mask.

MULTANI MITTI: Also known as Fuller's earth, it sucks out dirt from pores, is very rich in mineral content, and is used as a thickening and cleaning agent. For best results, apply after shower on a damp face. Rinse off once it dries thoroughly.

GRAPES: Being mildly acidic in nature, they act as a good cleaning and bleaching agent.

HENNA: As a coolant and skin dye, it has astringent and cosmetic properties.

LEMON: A rich source of pure, natural Vitamin C, it is used as a bleaching agent.

WATER MELON: Popularly known as *TARBOOJA*, it may be used to refresh and clean dry skin.

PUDINA: Also known as mint, it may be added to tea in digestive disorder. *Pudina* added to bath water is refreshing and stimulating.

ONION: To prevent blemishes, wash your face in onion juice. Mixed with honey, it acts as a natural anti-wrinkle and antiseptic lotion.

ORANGE PEEL: Dried and ground orange peel is used as a mask and facial scrub.

ROSE: This highly fragrant flower is the richest source of natural vitamin E or Youth vitamin. Ayurveda recommends *Roja Pushpa Avalehya* a semi solid (like *chyavanprasha*) to maintain youthfulness. This quenches thirst in summer and combats other related problems. *Gulkund* a sweet pan ingredient is made out of rose petals. This cools down the overworked body system.

STRAWBERRY: Being a rich source of iron, strawberry juice helps cleaning discoloured teeth, when used regularly.

SUGAR, SOAP AND LEMON: For an abrasive face scrub, lather the face with soap, then add a handful of sugar and scrub. Rinse off and finally apply lemon juice. This process thoroughly cleanses and stimulates the skin.

TEA: Due to its tannin content, it is soothing and healing as it absorbs ultra-violet light. It is used in sun tan creams to prevent burning. Teabags also make soothing eye pads.

SKIN AND VITAMINS

- **VITAMIN A** helps keep skin from drying out by helping circulation.
- **VITAMIN B** helps keep skin blemish-free.
- **VITAMIN C** purifies blood and helps keep you glowing. *Amla* and other citrus fruits are full of minerals and vitamin-C.
- **VITAMIN E** is the youthful vitamin helping keep skin young.
- Ample fresh fruits and vegetables, plenty of water and good, sound sleep provide natural nourishment to skin.

HERBALS IN SKIN CARE

- *SHATAVARI* (Asparagus racemoses) is one of the highly useful herbal drugs in skin care. The powder of the root 5 gm in quantity is taken orally with a cup of milk every evening to nourish dry skin and add lustre.
- **SILK COTTON TREE:** A paste made from the thorny skin of the silk cotton tree with milk, and applied removes black spots and brings lustre to the face.
- **FENUGREEK SEEDS (*METHI*):** The powder applied to the skin prevents dryness, roughness and coarseness.
- **COTTON SEED OIL:** It is a very useful dressing in clearing spots and freckles on the skin.
- **NUTMEG:** The local application of nutmeg paste (*jatiphala*) clears out white patches and blemishes on the skin.
- **CITRON AND COTUS:** A mixture of honey and the juice of citron (*bijora*) in which costus (*kustha*) has been sealed for a week is a useful cosmetic to keep skin soft.

HOME FACE MASKS

- **EGG WHITE MASK:** Beat the white of an egg and spread out as a thin film onto your face. Rinse off after 30 minutes. This mask lightens the skin and irons out wrinkles.

- **ONION MASK:** Mash and sieve an onion, mix onion juice with this into a paste and add 1 tablespoon of Fuller's earth and 1 teaspoon of honey. This mask prevents blemishes and wrinkles.

- **ALMOND MASK:** Mix 2 tablespoons ground almonds, one tablespoon rose water, 1/2 tablespoon honey into a paste and apply onto the face. Leave on for 20 minutes and rinse off.

HAIR AND HERBS

- **BITTER ALMONDS** are made into a paste and applied on the scalp, regularly to get rid of dandruff and hair lice.
- **EGG YOLK** is an excellent conditioner for dry hair.
- **HENNA** is a natural hair dye with astringent and cooling properties.
- **TOBACCO AND *RITHA*:** Apply the mixture of tobacco powder and water, keep on for 2-3 hours followed by washing with an emulsion of soapnut (*ritha*).
- **YOGHURT:** Applied to the hair it is a good remedy for dandruff.

HOME MADE SHAMPOOS

- **EGG SHAMPOO:** Eggs are rich sources of proteins. Beat 2 egg yolks into a glass of hot water. Strain. Soak hair and scalp in this solution for an hour. Rinse off with warm water.

- **HERBAL SHAMPOO:** Add 100 gram each of dried *ritha* and *amla* to one litre of water and soak for 24 hours. Boil and allow to cool. Strain and use as a shampoo to bring silky smoothness and tonicity to hair.

- **SOFT SHAMPOO:** Wash 150 gm each of dried clives and *shikakai* leaves in cold water and soak overnight in an iron pot. The next morning, these are tested for 10-15 minutes and strained. Liquidise the remaining pulp and use the paste to wash your hair for a soft and shiny look.

177

GENERAL HAIR CARE

Every woman's secret desire is to make her crowning glory a healthy asset to her personality. Here's how to keep those silky stands healthy and happy.

DIET: Requirements for healthy hair are:
1. Balanced diet: Preferably rich in a protein called keratin.
2. Fatty acids, minerals and vitamins especially iron, zinc, vitamin C and B complex.
   This includes egg, cheese, meat, fish, whole grains, nuts and green vegetables.

CLEANING: Regular washing is necessary to keep your hair looking and feeling good. Use a shampoo that suits your hair type and avoid using hot water on your scalp. Use warm or cool water.

Everytime you wash your hair apply shampoo twice and lather, rinsing after each application. Gently massage the shampoo onto your scalp. Rinse the soap off completely. For the final rinse, add a little vinegar to the water to remove soap and leave hair soft and shiny. Yoghurt is also a good natural conditioner. You may massage yoghurt onto your hair and scalp for 5 minutes before rinsing off.

BRUSHING: Apart from keeping your hair clean, regular combing and brushing is necessary to remove dirt and dust and to stimulate circulation. Gently brush your head and hair everyday so that the scalp gets a mild massage.

Make sure your brushes have soft rounded bristles so that they do not pull your hair and damage it.

Wash your brushes with a little shampoo and an old toothbrush everytime you wash your hair.

IDENTIFYING YOUR HAIR TYPE

Generally your hair type is similar to your skin type i.e. if your skin is greasy, it is likely that your hair is greasy too. Your lifestyle and diet reflect on your hair and skin to some extent.

NORMAL HAIR is usually shiny and healthy, ideally, it should be washed once a week.

DRY HAIR looks dull with dry splitends. If your diet contains enough zinc and fatty acids and if you wash your hair with a mild shampoo once a week, it would help relieve dryness. You could also wash it with a nourishing egg shampoo.

Warm oil massages are most beneficial. Avoid subjecting hair to perms and dyes.

GREASY HAIR becomes lank and can leave the forehead greasy. Avoid greasy and fried food. Eat plenty of green and fresh vegetables. Drink plenty of water and fruit juices. Wash hair twice a week and add lemon juice to the final rinse. You can also try a massage with *neem* oil.

DANDRUFF can affect all skin types and is a common problem. Regular washing, combing, brushing plus a balanced diet helps in preventing it. A hot steam bath can combat dandruff. Massage hot oil onto your scalp and wrap a hot damp towel around your head. You may reapply towels until 30 minutes.

LIFESTYLE

The condition of your hair can vary according to climate, diet and changes in your lifestyle. If you feel your hair is dull or falling more than usual, check your lifestyle. Are you worried and stressed out? Overworked? Eating too much of junk food? Not getting enough rest? Even illness, medication and hormonal changes affect your hair. So it is better to change habits rather than a shampoo.

5. SIMPLE HOME MEDICAL TESTS

The number of people using home medical kits to detect signs of imminent ill-health or pregnancy is on the rise. (Thanks to advancement of technology and simplification of usage, it has made life easier for a lot of busy people, who need not waste precious time running to laboratories and awaiting results).

This is of course not to encourage self diagnosis or self-treatment but to help determine whether and when to see a doctor.

Some of the commonly used medical kits are listed below:

1. **Pregnancy Test Kit:** This test determines the presence of a hormone called HCG (Human chorionic gonadotropin) in the urine of the woman. This is one of the most widely used home medical kits.

2. **Ovulation Test Kit:** This test detects the presence of another hormone LH (Luteinizing Hormone) which is present in the urine of the woman just one day prior to her ovulation. This is widely used in the area of infertility.

3. **Blood Glucose Test/Diabetic Test Kit:** This has grown to be a very popular and useful kit for diabetics, who until recently were harrowed with endless visits to the lab to determine their blood glucose levels.

    This test is determined by applying a drop of blood to a strip of plastic (the tip of which is paper treated with a chemical) and then matching the column on the strip with a given colour chart. Another method requires insertion of the strip into an electronic meter with a digital display of the blood sugar level.

4. **Blood Pressure Apparatus:** This has become a very common household commodity and is available both in the traditional mercurial as well as the modern display models. The readings may be taken from the arm, wrist or a finger even.

Though the above are the most commonly used apparatus at home, there are other test kits to determine various physical conditions including leukocytosis, haemorrhoids (piles), ulcers, high blood cholesterol and even tuberculosis, hepatitis and AIDS.

Still it is suggested that any positive finding be counter-checked at the laboratory and reported to a physician as early as possible to avoid delay in diagnosis and treatment.

HOUSEHOLD POISONS

Many substances found in a normal household are poisonous and are likely to cause harm, if improperly stored, especially to children.

POISONS: These include:

1. Liquid soap 2. Some cosmetics 3. Fire lighters 4. Turpentine 5. Bleach 6. Rat Poison 7. Paints 8. Garden sprays 9. Insecticides etc.

The symptoms and signs may vary according to the poison, although vomiting and abdominal pain are likely to occur in most cases.

MANAGEMENT

- Rush the victim to a hospital at once.
- Send any samples of vomit and containers such as bottles or pill boxes found nearby to the hospital with the casualty.
- Children are also liable to take medicines and tablets, colourful capsules found in the house. While most household medicines are not dangerous if taken as directed, many are poisonous if the dosage is exceeded.

CAUTION

Always make sure that all bottles and jars containing poisonous substances are neatly marked and kept out of the reach of children.

Part-IV
Glossary

1. GLOSSARY OF AYURVEDIC STANDARD MEDICINES AND THEIR MANUFACTURES

Complaint	Drugs
1. ABDOMINAL PAIN	a. *Shankha Vati* (Baidyanath) 1 tablet thrice a day. b. *Pudin Hara* (Dabur) 1 tablet thrice a day. c. *Kumaryasava* (Baidyanath, Zandu, Dabur) 15 ml with equal quantity of water. d. *Bhaskara Lavana* (Dabur, Baidyanath) 2 gm with buttermilk. **Note:** To be avoided by hypertensive patients. e. *Amadoshantak Capsules* (Jamma Pharmacy) 1 capsule twice a day. f. *Rason Zyme* (Deen Dayal Aushad, Gwalior) 1 capsule twice a day.
2 ABORTION (THREATENING)	a. *Phala Kalyana Ghritam* (Baidyanath) 5ml twice a day mixed in a cup of hot milk. b. *Meryton Syrup* (Vasu) 2 to 3 tsf thrice a day c. Leptaden (Alarsin) 2 tablets thrice a day continuously fo 3 months.
3. ABSCESS	a. *Septillin* (Himalaya Drug Co.) 1 tablet thrice a day. b. *Kanchanara Guggulu* (Zandu) 1 tablet thrice a day. c. *Saribadyasavam* (Baidyanath) 15 ml with equal quantity of water. d. *Cutfar Ointment* (BAN) Ext. application. e. *Step Caps* (Vasu) 1 capsule thrice a day.
4. ACIDITY	a. *Sooktyn* (Alarsin) 1 tablet thrice a day with fruit juice/milk. b. *Kamadudha Rasa* (Plain) (Zandu, Dabur) 2 pills twice a day.

183

Complaint	Drugs
	c. *Avipattikara Choorna* (Baidyanath) 3 gm with lukewarm water twice a day.
	d. *Drakshadi Lehyam* (Dabur) 1 teaspoon twice a day with milk.
	e. *Alsarex* (Charak) 1 tablet thrice a day.
	f. *Acidinol* (BAN) 1 tablet thrice a day.
	g. *Soota Sekhar* (Sandu) 1 tablet twice a day.
	h. *Avipattikara Churna* (Zandu) ½ tsf twice a day with Lukewarm water.
	i. *Plantacid* (Phyto) *Caps.* 1 capsule twice a day.
5. ACNE	a. *Raktashodhan* (Baidyanath) 1 tablet twice a day.
	b. *R.S. Forte Syrup* (DAP) 2 tablespoons twice a day.
	c. *Septillin* (Himalaya Drug Co.) 1 tab. twice a day.
	d. *Kumkumadi Lepam* (IMPCOPS, Chennai) to be applied locally.
	e. *Safi* (Hamdard) 2 tsf twice a day.
	f. *Hema Pushpa* (Raj Vaidya Co.) 1 tablet twice a day.
	g. *Neemayu* (Yash Ramedes) (MP) 1 tablet twice a day
	h. *Acnovin* (Vasu) Crean for Ext. application.
	i. *R.S.Fort.* (Bajaj) *Syrup* 3 tsp twice a day.
6. ALLERGY (RESPIRATORY)	a. *Chitraka Haritaki Lehyam* (Dabur/Zandu) with water.
	b. *Vasarishta* (Baidyanath/Zandu/Dabur) 15 ml with equal quantity of water.
	c. *Dekofcyn* (Alarsin) 1 tablet thrice a day.
	d. *Crux Syrup* (BAN) 1 tsp as required.
	e. *Drill Syrup* (BAN) 1 tsp thrice a day.
	f. *Chitraka Hareetaki* (Dabur) 1 tsf twice a day.
7. ALLERGY (SKIN)	a. *Brihad Haridra Khanda* (Baidyanath) 5gms twice a day with milk or hot water.
	b. *Laghu Sutasekhara Vati* (Baidyanath) 2 pills twice a day.
	c. *Triphala Choorna* (Dabur) 5gm with lukewarm water at bedtime.
	d. *Dermasyl Ointment* (Sahaj) for ext. applications
	e. *Dermafax Soap* (BAN) for Regular bath.
	f. *Radona Tab.* and *Syrup* (Solumiks) 1 tab. twice a day 2 tsf twice a day.

Complaint	Drugs
8. AMENORRHOEA	a. *Aloe Compound* (Alarsin) 2 tablets twice a day. b. *Aloes Compound* (Alarsin) 2 tablets twice a day 3 months. c. *Senovila* (Solumiks) 1 tab. twice a day
9. AMOEBIASIS	a. *Amoebica* (Baidyanath) 1 tablet thrice a day. b. *Kutaja Tablets* (DAP) 1 tablet twice a day. c. *Bilva Avaleham* (Baidyanath/Zandu) 1 teaspoon twice a day. d. *Antisar Cap.* (Chandrika) 1 cap. twice a day. e. *Mebarid* (Phyto Pharma) 1 cap. twice a day.
10. ANAEMIA	a. *Heamol* (Sandu) 2 tablets twice a day. b. *Mandoora Vataka* (Zandu) 2 pills twice a day. c. *Raktoj Syrup* (Bajaj) 15 ml twice a day. d. *Lohasavam* (Baidyanath) 15 ml twice a day. e. *Limiron Granules* (Phyto Pharma) 1 tablespoon twice a day with milk. f. *Feroliv-Forte* (BAN) 1 cap. twice a day with milk after food. g. *Raktoj* (Bajaj) Syrup 4 tsf twice a day. h. *Wranger* (BAN) 15ml twice a day. i. *Efiplus Caps.* (Solumiks) 1 cap. twice a day.
11. APPETITE-LOSS	a. *Sitopaladi Churna* (Zandu) 1 teaspoon with water (Note. Contra-indicated in diabetics). b. *Draksharishta* (Baidyanath) 15 ml twice a day. c. *Pudin-Hara* (Dabur) 1 pellet twice a day. d. *Lashunadi Vati* (Baidyanath) 1 tab. twice a day. e. *Limiron Granules* (Phyto Pharma) 1 tablespoon twice a day with milk. f. *Feroliv-forte* (BAN) 1 cap. twice a day with mild after food. g. *Raktoj* (Bajaj) Syrup 4 tsf twice a day. h. *Wranger* (BAN) 15ml twice a day. i. *Efiplus Caps.* (Solumiks) 1 cap. twice a day.
12. ARTHRITIS (A) ARTHRITIS RHEUMATOID	a. *Amavatari Ras* (Baidyanath/Dabur) 1 tablet twice a day. b. *R. Compound* (Alarsin) 2 tablets twice a day. c. *Maha Rasnadi Kada* (Baidyanath) 15 ml twice a day. d. *Rumadap Oil* (DAP) for external application.

Complaint	Drugs
	e. *R. Compound* (Alarsin) 2 tablet twice a day.
	f. *R. Pairyn* (BAN) 2 tablets twice a day.
	g. *Rheumat-90* (Nagarjuna, Kerala) 15ml twice a day.
	h. *Rasonzyme Caps.* (Deendayal, Gwalior) 1 cap. twice a day.
	i. *Rheumasyl Linement* (Zandu) (For ext. application).
	j. *Arnopen Caps.* (Phytopharma) 1 cap. twice a day.
(B) OSTEOARTHRITIS	a. *Stresscom Capsules* (Dabur) 1 capsule twice a day.
	b. *Rumayog* (Zandu) one tablet thrice a day.
	c. *Chyavan Yog* (Bajaj) 1 tablespoon twice a day.
	d. *Maha Masha Tailam* (Baidyanath) for external application.
	e. *Remorin* (J & J Dechane) 2 caps. twice a day.
	f. *Dazzle Caps.* (Vasu) 1 cap. thrice a day.
	g. *Painoff Oil* (Jain) for external use only.
	h. *Rhue Oil* (Ban) for external use only.
	i. *Myostal Tablets* (Soluniks) 1 tab. twice a day.
13. ASTHMA (BRONCHIAL)	a. *Broncap* (Capro) 1 capsule twice a day with hot water.
	b. *Spasma* (Charak) *Syrup* 3 teaspoons twice a day.
	c. *Vasa Kantakari Lehyam* (Zandu/Baidyanath) one teaspoon twice a day with warm water.
	d. *Branco Cap.* (Capro) 1 cap. twice a day.
	e. *Zeal cap.* (Vasu) 1 cap. twice a day.
14. ATHEROSCLEROSIS	a. *Guggulip* (Cipla) one tablet twice a day.
	b. *Garlip* (Phytopharma) 2 tablets twice a day.
	c. *Yogaraja Guggulu* (Zandu) 1 tablet twice a day.
15. AGREESSIVE BEHAVIOUR	a. *Mentat Tabs.* (Himalaya) 2 tablets twice a day.
	b. *Manasa Mitra Vatakam* (AVS) 1 tab. twice a day.
	c. *Brahmi Vati* (Dabur) 1 tab. thrice a day.
16. ALBUMINURIA	a. *K_4 Tabs.* 2 tabs. twice a day.
	b. *Chandamadi Vati* (Baidyanath) 1 tab. twice a day.
	c. *Bangshil* (Alarsin) tabs 1 tab. thrice a day.
17. ANAL FISTULA	a. *Triphala Guggul* (Zandu) 2 tabs. thrice a day.
	b. *Pilex Ointment* (Himalaya) Local application.
	c. *Saribadi Vati* (Baidyanath) 2 tabs. twice a day.

Complaint	Drugs
18. ANGINA PECTORISIS	a. *Abana* (Himalaya) 2 tabs. twice a day. b. *Jawahar Mohar No. 1* (Zandu) 1 pill twice a day. c. *Arjun Tabs.* (Chrak) 1 tab. thrice a day.
19. ANXIETY	a. *Siledin* (Alarsin) 2 tabs. twice a day. b. *Brento Tabs.* (Zandu) 1 tab. thrice a day. c. *Gerifort Tabs.* (Himalaya) 2 tabs. twice a day. d. *Brahmi Vati* (Dabur) 1 tab. twice a day.
20. BACKACHE	a. *Sallaki Tablet* (Gufic) 1 tablet twice a day. b. *Rumayog* (Zandu) 1 tablet twice a day. c. *Stressnil* (Baidyanath) 1 tablet twice a day. d. *Rumalaya* (Himalaya) cream for external application. e. *Rhymasyl* (Zandu) ointment for external application. f. *Myron* (Alarsin) *Tabs.* Females only 2 tabs. twice a day. g. *Pyroflex Linament/Gel* (Soluniks) apply on the affected area.
21. BALD HEAD	a. *Hair-Rich Oil* (Capro) local application (to be rubbed on the affected area). b. *Bhringaraja Asava* (Dabur) 15 ml with equal quantity of water twice a day.
22. BED SORES	a. *Tankana* (Baidyanath) to be sprinkled on the sores after cleaning and drying. b. *Septillin* (Himalaya) 1 tablet thrice a day. c. *R.S. Forte Syrup* (DAP) 2 teaspoons twice a day.
23. BED-WETTING	a. *Shilajit Capsules* (Dabur) 1 capsule twice a day. b. *Chandraprabha Vati* (Zandu/Baidyanath) 1 tablet twice a day.
24. BLEEDING GUMS	a. *Gum Tone* (Charak) to be applied on gums. b. *G-32 Tab.* (Alarsin) 1 tablet crushed and applied over gums twice daily. c. *Amalaki Rasayana* (Baidyanath) 3g twice a day d. *Vasa Ghana Vati* (Chaitanya) 1 tablet twice a day. e. *Charmon Drops* (BAN, Rajkol) 10 to 15 drops twice a day (Children). f. *Amlaki Ghanvati* (Chaitanya) 2 tabs. thrice a day. g. *Chavan Cap.* (Capro) 1 cap. thrice a day. h. *Styplon Tab.* (Himalaya) 2 tabs. twice a day. i. *Gum Tone* (Powder) (Charak) to be applied on the gums thrice a day.

Complaint	Drugs
25. BODY ACHES/PAIN	a. *Rumalaya* (Himalaya) one tablet twice a day.
	b. *Godanti Misrama* (Baidyanath) 1 tablet twice a day.
	c. *Rumayog* (Zandu) 1 tablet twice a day.
	d. *Pain Off Tabs.* (Jain) 1 tab. thrice a day.
	e. *Myostal Tabs.* (Soluniks) 1 tab. thrice a day.
	f. *Sallaki Tabs.* (Gufic) 1 tab. twice a day.
	g. *Remorin Caps.* (J&J Dechane) 1 tab. thrice a day.
26. BRONCHITIS	a. *Broncap* (Capro) 1 capsule twice a day.
	b. *Lakshmivilas Ras* (Dabur/Zandu) 1 tablet twice a day.
	c. *Sitopaladi Choorna* (Dabur) 5 gm with honey.
	d. *Chitraka Hareetaki* (Dabur) 1 teaspoonful twice a day.
	e. *Decofcyn Syrup* (Alarsin) 2 teaspoonful as required.
	f. *Hemoplex Tab.* (J&J Dechane) 1 tab twice a day.
27. BURNS	a. *Sapta Guna Tailam* (Baidyanath) for external application.
	b. *Dermodap* (DAP) for external application.
	c. *Triphala Guggul* (Zandu) twice a day.
	d. *Manjista Kada* (Zandu) 15 ml twice a day.
	e. *Ripanto Ointment* (J&J Dechane) for ext. application.
	f. *Epderm Capsules* (Capro) 1 cap. twice a day.
28. BREAST (UNDER-DEVELOPMENT)	a. *Shatavarex* (Zandu) *Granules* 2 teaspoonful twice a day with milk.
29. BREASTMILK (TO IMPROVE)	a. *Leptaden* (Alarsin) 2 tabs. twice a day with milk.
	b. *Shatavarex Granules* (Zandu) 1 teaspoonful twice a day.
30. BURNING URINE	a. *K4 Tablet* (Zandu) 2 tabs. twice a day.
	b. *Bangshil* (Alarsin) tabs. 2 tabs twice a day.
	c. *Chandanadivati* (Baidyanath) 1 tablet twice a day.
	d. *Gokshuru Kada* (Sando) 2 teaspoonful twice a day.
31. CARBUNCLE DIABETIC	a. *Septillin* (Himalaya) 1 tablet twice a day.
	b. *Kanchanara Guggulu* (Zandu) 1 tablet twice a day.
32. CERVICAL SPONDYLOSIS	a. *Ksheerabala Capsules* (AVS Kottakkal) 1 capsule twice a day.
	b. *Sallaki Plus* (Gufic) 1 tablet twice a day.
	c. *Rumasyl Cream* (Zandu) for external application.

Complaint	Drugs
	d. *Rhumayog* (Zandu) tabs 2 tablet twice a day.
	e. *Rasnadi guggul* (Nagarjuna Kerala) 1 tablet thrice a day.
	f. *Pain Off Tabs.* (Jain) 1 tablet thrice a day.
	g. *Dazzle Cap.* (Vasu) 1 capsule twice a day.
	h. *Remorin* (J&J Dechame) 2 capsule thrice a day.
33. CIRRHOSIS OF LIVER	a. *Stimliv* (Franco-Indian) 2 tablets twice a day.
	b. *Jaundex Syrup* (Sandu) 10 ml twice a day.
	c. *Arogyavardhini Vati* (Zandu) 1 tablet twice a day.
	d. *Cytozen* (Charak) 1 tablet twice daily.
34. COMMON COLD	a. *Trishun* (Zandu) 1 tablet twice a day.
	b. *F.15* (DAP) 1 tablet twice a day.
	c. *Plug it Cap.* (Vasu) 1 capsule twice a day.
	d. *Halin Drops* (Nargarjuna, Kerala) sprinkle 2 to 3 drops on a towel and inhale frequently.
	e. *Cold Vin Tabs.* (Yash Ramadas Amdavad) 1 tab. thrice a day.
	f. *Laxmivilas Ras* (Dabur) 1 tab. twice a day.
35. CONJUNCTIVITIS	a. *I-tone* (Dey's) *Eye Drops* 1-2 drops repeatedly in both eyes.
	b. *Biogest* (Kerala Ayurvedic Pharmacy) one tablet twice a day.
	c. *Opthocare Eye Drops* (Himalaya) 3 to 4 drops to be applied in both the eyes thrice a day.
	d. *Triphala Churna* (Dabur) 1 teaspoonful at bed-time with warm water.
	e. *Triphala Grutham* (Baidyanath) 1 tsf twice a day with warm milk.
36. CONSTIPATION	a. *Herbolax* (Himalaya) 1 tablet at bedtime.
	b. *Deendayal Churna* (Shankar Pharmacy) 1 tablespoon at bedtime with hot water.
	c. *Lion Churna* (Narnarayan) 1 tablespoon at bedtime.
	d. *Kayam Churna* (Sheth Bros.) 1 tablespoon with lukewarm water at bed-time.
	e. *Suprabhat Powder (Tan Sukh)* 1 tablespoon at bed-time with hot water.
	f. *Triphala Churna* (Dabur) 1 teaspoon at bed-time with lukewarm water.

Complaint	Drugs
37. COUGH (DRY)	a. *Yashti Choorna* (Zandu) 3gm with lukewarm milk. b. *Kantakari Tablet* (Chaitanya) 1 tablet twice a day. c. *Supress Cough Syrup* (Nagarjuna Kerala) 3 tablespoons thrice a day. d. *Dekofcyn Tablet* (Alarsin) 1 tablet thrice a day. e. *Laxmi Vilas* (Dabur) 1 tab. twice a day with honey. f. *Kofol Tablet* (Charak) 1 tab. thrice a day. g. *Crux Syrup* (BAN) 2 teaspoons thrice a day.
38. COUGH (PRODUCTIVE)	a. *Tulsi Cough Syrup* (Bajaj, DAP) 2 teaspoons thrice a day. b. *Vasaka* (Sandu) 2 tablespoons thrice a day. c. *Decofsyn Tablet* (Alarsin) 1 tablet thrice a day. d. *Kasni Syrup* (Malarul) 2 teaspoons twice a day. e. *Hookuf Syrup* (Madan (up)) 1 to 2 teaspoons twice a day. f. *Ela Deshamoola Lehyam* (Nagarjuna Karala) 1 to 3 grams twice a day. g. *Sitophaladi Churna* (Dabur) 1/2 tablespoon twice a day.
39. CRAMPS	a. *Sallaki* (Gufic) 1 tablet thrice a day. b. *R. Compound* (Alarsin) 2 tablets twice a day. c. *Rumalaya Cream* (Himalaya) for external application. d. *Myostal Tabs. & Oil* (Solmukis) 2 tablets twice a day. Oil or massage on the affected part. e. *Rhumayog* (Zandu) *Tabs.* 2 tablets twice a day. f. *Stress-Com* (Dabur) 1 cap. twice a day.
40. CRACKS (FEET)	a. *Dermodap Ointment* (DAP) for external application b. *Pinda Tailam* (Arya Vaidyasala Kottakkal) for external application. c. *Healex Ointment* (Baidyanath) for external application d. *Sindooradi Lepan* (IMIS) for external application. e. *Manjista Kada* (Baidyanath) 15ml thrice a day. f. *Neem Ayu Tab.* (Yash) 1 tablet twice a day.
41. CUTS	a. *Saptaguna Tailam* (Baidyanath) for external application. b. *Saptamruta Loha* (Zandu) 1 tab twice a day.
42. DANDRUFF	a. *Durdura Patradi Tailam* (AVS, Kottakal) or *Durvadi Tailam* (IMPCOPS) for external application. b. *Epderm* (Capro) *Caps.* 1 cap. twice daily.

Complaint	Drugs
	c. *Oil 777* (Siddha) for ext. application into scalp.
	d. *Aarogya Vardani* (Zandu) ½ tablet twice a day for 10 days.
	e. *R.S. Forte Syrup* (Bajaj) 2 teaspoons twice a day.
	f. *Brahmivati* (Dabur) 1 tab. twice a day.
43. DEPRESSION	a. *Stress Com* (Dabur) 1 capsule twice a day.
	b. *Drakshojem* (DAP) 15 ml twice daily.
	c. *Siledin Tabs.* (Alarsin) 1 tablet twice a day.
	d. *Memorin Capsule* (Phyto) 1 capsule twice a day.
	f. *Brentrex Capsule* (Anuja) 1 capsule twice a day.
44. DIABETES (As a supplement only)	a. *Diabecon* (Himalaya) 2 tablets twice a day.
	b. *Hyponid* (Charak) 1 tablet twice daily.
	c. *Nishamlaki* (IMPCOPS) 2 tablets twice a day.
	d. *Mersina* (J & J Dechane) 2 tablets twice a day.
	e. *Gluco Dap* (Bajaj) *Capsule* 1 capsule twice a day.
	f. *JK 22 Tablet* (Charak) 1 tablet twice a day.
	g. *Madu Mardan Powder* (Jain) 1 tablespoon once a day.
45. DIARRHOEA	a. *Kutja Tab.* (DAP) 2 tablets twice a day.
	b. *Karpooradi Vati* (Zandu) (without opium) 2 tablets twice a day.
	c. *Pudin Hara* for children (Dabur) 1 tablet twice a day.
	d. *Berbenterone Syrup* (Sandu) 1 tablespoon thrice daily.
	e. *Deepan* (Charak) 1 tablet twice daily.
	f. *Diarex Tabs.* (Himalaya) 2 tablets twice a day.
46. DYSENTERY	a. *Mebarid Tablet* (Phyto Pharma) 1 tablet twice a day.
	b. *Amoebica Tablet* (Baidyanath) 1 tablet twice a day.
	c. *Bilvavalehyam* (Sandu) 1 teaspoon twice a day.
	d. *Kutaj Tabs.* (DAP) 1 tablet thrice a day.
	e. *Berbenterome Pediatric syrup* (Sandu) 1 teaspoon thrice a day. (for children)
	f. *Ambimap Tablets* (Maharshi) 1 tab thrice a day.
47. DYSFUNCTIONAL UTERINE BLEEDING (DUB)	a. *Vasa Ghana Vati* (Chaitanya) 1 tablet twice a day.
	b. *Ayopan* (Alarsin) 2 tablets twice a day.
	c. *M2 Tone* (Charak) 1 tablet twice a day.
	d. *M2 Tone Syrup* 2 teaspoons thrice a day.

Complaint	Drugs
	e. *Posex Fort Tabs.* (Charak) 2 tablets thrice a day.
	f. *Ashatone Tabs. & Syrup* (Dhootpape) 2 tabs twice a day. Syrup 4 teaspoons twice a day.
48. DYSMENORRHOEA	a. *Aloe Compound* (Alarsin) 2 tablets twice a day starting 3 days before expected date of menses.
	b. *Pathyadi Quatha* (Sandu) 15 ml twice a day.
	c. *Menocramp Tab.* (Solmuks) 1 tab twice a day.
	d. *Plug-it Caps.* (Vasu) 1 capsule twice a day.
	e. *Utrodap* (DAP) 2 tablets twice a day.
	f. *Kumari Asavam* (Dabur) 3 tablespoons thrice a day.
	g. *Pavioff Tabs.* (Java) 1 tablet twice a day.
	h. *Dashamoolarishtha* (abu) 3 tablespoons twice a day.
49. DIARRHOEA	a. *Diarex Tabs.* (Himalaya) 1 tab thrice a day.
	b. *Kutaj Tabs.* (Bajaj) 1 tablet thrice a day.
	c. *Karpooradi Vati* (Zandu) 2 pills thrice a day.
	d. *Pudina Hara* (Dabur)
	e. *Mebarid Capsule* (Phyto) 1 capsule thrice a day.
	f. *Deepan Tabs.* (Chark) 1 tablet thrice a day.
50. EAR-ACHE	a. *Kshara Tail Ear Drops* (Baidyanath) 3 to 4 drops to be instilled in the ears.
	b. *Saribadivati* (Baidyanath) 1 tablet thrice a day with water.
51. ECZEMA	a. *Pancha Tikta Grutha Guggulu* (Zandu) 2 teaspoons with hot milk/water on empty stomach.
	b. *Epderm Capsules* (Capro) 1 capsule twice a day.
	c. *Dermodap* (DAP) ointment for external application only.
	d. *Cutis Caps.* (Vasu) 1 capsule twice a day.
	e. *Dermasyl Ointment* (Sahaj) for ext. use application.
	f. *R.S. Syrup* (Bajaj) 2 teaspoons twice a day.
	g. *Aarogyavardini* (Zandu) 1 tablet twice a day.
	h. *Brahmivati* (Baidyanath) 1 tablet twice a day.
52. EOSINOPHILIA	a. *Kantakari Tabs.* (Chaitanya) 2 tablets twice a day.
	b. *Lohasavam* (Baidyanath) 3 teaspoons twice a day.
	c. *Chitraka Hareetati* (Dabur) 1 teaspoon twice a day.
53. FATIGUE	a. *Stress Nil Caps.* (Baidyanath) 1 capsule twice a day with milk.

Complaint	Drugs

b. *Stress Com Caps.* (Dabur) 1 capsule twice a day with milk.
c. *Wranger* (Vasu) 2 teaspoons thrice a day.
d. *Albosan* (J&J Dechane) *Tablet* 2 tabs. twice a day.
e. *Fortege Tab.* (Alarsin) 2 teaspoons twice a day.
f. *Alpitone Liq.* (Zandu) 2 teaspoons twice a day.
g. *Monoll* (Charak) 2 teaspoons twice a day.
h. *Afrodet Caps.* (Soluniks) 1 capsule twice a day.

54. FROZEN SHOULDER
a. *Sallaki* (GUFIC) 1 tablet thrice a day.
b. *Remorin Cap.* (J&J Dechare) 1 capsule thrice a day.
c. *Rheumasyl* (Zandu) ointment for ext. application.
d. *Myostal Tabs.* (Solumiks) 1 tablet thrice a day.

55. FEVER
a. *Chirakin* (Zandu) *Tabs.* 2 tablets twice a day.
b. *Antimal* (Bajaj) *Tabs.* 2 tablets twice a day.
c. *Painoff* (Jain) *Tabs.* 1 tablet twice a day.

56. FACIAL PALSY
a. *Rasonzyme Caps.* (Deendayal) 1 cap twice a day.
b. *Rhumadap* (Bajaj) 2 tablets twice a day.
c. *Stress Com Caps.* (Dabur).

57. GASTRITIS
a. *Sooktyn Tablet* (Alarsin) 1 tablet twice a day.
b. *Soota Sekhar Ras* 1 tablet twice a daily.

58. HEAD-ACHE
a. *Godanti Mishran* (Baidyanath) 2 pills twice a day.
b. *Pain off Tablets* (Jain) 1 tablet twice a day.
c. *Feroonil Tab.* (Ahuja) 1 tablet thrice a day.
d. *Cephagran* (Charak) 1 tab thrice a day.
e. *Sirashoola Vajaratak Ras* (Baidyanath) 2 pills twice a day.

59. HYSTERIA
a. *Ashwagandharishta* (Zandu) 15 ml twice a day with equal quantity of water.
b. *Serpina* (Himalya) *Tabs.* 1 tablet twice a day.
c. *Albosang Tab.* (J&J) 2 tabs twice a day.
d. *Stressnil Cap.* (Baidyanath) 1 capsule twice a day.
e. *Saraswatha Gruitha* (Nagarjuna) 2 teaspoons twice a day with warm milk.

60. HALITOSIS (Bad Breath)
a. *Triphala Kada* (Sandu) 15 ml twice a day.
b. *Eladi Gutika* (Baidyanath) 1 tablet to be chewed thrice a day.
c. *Kadiradi Bati* (Dabur) 1 tab. thrice a day.
d. *Salphos Tabs.* (J&J Dechane) 2 tabs. twice a day.

Complaint	Drugs
61. HOARSE-VOICE	a. *Yasti Madhu Churna* (Zandu) 1 teaspoon twice a day with warm milk. b. *Kadiradi Bati* (Dabur) chew 1 to 6 tabs. a day.
62. HIGH BP (Hypertension)	a. *Jessica Tabs.* (IMIS) 2 tablets thrice a day. b. *Serpina* (Himalaya) 2 tablets twice a day. c. *Brento Tabs.* (Zandu) 2 tablets twice a day.
63. INFLUENZA	a. *F.15 Tablets* 1 tablet thrice a day. b. *Sudarshana Ghana Vati* 1 tablet twice a day. c. *Corazan Cap.* (Zandu) 1 capsule twice a day. d. *Antimal Tab.* (Bajaj) 2 tablets twice a day. e. *Chirakin* (Zandu) *Tab.* 1 tablet thrice a day. f. *Laxmivilas Ras* (Dabur) 1 tab. twice a day.
64. INTESTINAL WORMS	a. *Vidangarista* (Baidyanath) 15 ml twice a day with equal water. b. *Wormahal Tabs.* (Aruja) 1 tablet twice a day. c. *Krumigna Vadika* (Nagarjuna Kerala) 1 tablet twice a day.
65. JAUNDICE	a. *Jaundex Syrup* (Sandu) 15 ml thrice a day. b. *Crytozen* (Charak) 1 tablet twice a day. c. *Liv-52 Drops* (Himalaya) six drops thrice a day for children. d. *Stimliv* (Franco) 2 tablets twice a day. e. *Hepajaum Caps.* 1 cap. twice a day. f. *Nirocil Tab.* (Solink) 2 tablets twice a day. g. *Livomap Tab. Syrup* (Maharshi) 2 tsf twice a day.
66. KIDNEY (URINARY) STONES	a. *Patherina* (Baidyanath) 1 tablet twice a day with a glass of water. b. *Cystone Tabs.* (Himalaya) 2 tablets twice a day. c. *Neeri Tabs.* (Almi-Delhi) 2 tabs. twice a day. d. *Stonvil Caps.* (Phyto) 1 capsule twice a day.
67. LEUCODERMA	a. *Aarogyavardini Tablets* (Zandu) 1 tablet twice daily. b. *Amlaki Rasayanam* (Baidyanath) 5 gms twice a day. c. *Pigmento Tabs.* (Charak) 2 tabs. twice a day. d. *Epderm Caps.* (Capro) 1 cap. twice a day. e. *Lid Oil* (Ayu. Lab., Rajkot) for ext. application.
68. LEUCORRHOEA	a. *Lukol* (Himalaya) 2 tablets twice a day. b. *Myron* (Alarsin) 1 tablet twice a day.

Complaint	Drugs
	c. *Lodhrasava* (Baidyanath) 15 ml twice a day.
	d. *Femigen* (Phyto) *Caps.* 1 capsule twice a day.
	e. *Lumital Tab.* (Solunik) 1 tablet twice a day.
	f. *Femiplex* (Charak) 2 tablet twice a day.
	g. *Albosang Tabs.* (J&J Dechana) 1 tab. thrice a day.
69. LOSS OF HAIR	a. *Trich-up Hair Oil* (For ext. application).
	b. *Kesha Kant Tablet* (Shankar) 1 tablet twice a day.
	c. *Keshranjana* (Aagom) *Oil* and *Tab.* 1 tablet twice a day. Oil to be applied on the head.
	d. *Kesh Sarita Oil* (Yash Remedies) used as hair oil.
	e. *Sesa Oil* (BAN) used as regular hair oil.
	f. *Hair Rich Caps.* (BAN) 1 capsule twice a day.
70. LOW B.P.	a. *Stress Com. Capsule* 1 capsule twice a day.
	b. *Drakshojem* (Bajaj) 15 ml twice a day with equal water.
	c. *Restora* (Dabur) 2 tablespoons thrice a day.
	d. *Sidda Makhara Dwaja* (Dabur) 1 tablet twice a day.
	e. *A.G. Fort* (Bajaj) 1 tablespoon thrice a day.
71. MALARIA	a. *Sudarshana Ghana Vati* (Baidyanath) 2 pills twice a day.
	b. *Antimal Tablets* (DAP) 2 tablets thrice a day.
	c. *Feronil Tabs.* (Anuja) 2 tablets thrice a day.
	d. *Chirakin* (Zandu) *Tabs.* 1 tablet thrice a day.
	e. *Amrutarista* (Dabur) 4 teaspoons thrice a day.
72. MEASLES	a. *Nirocil Tabs.* (Solmuki) 1 tab twice a day.
	b. *Antimal Tablets* (DAP) 2 tabs thrice a day.
	c. *Neem Ayu. Tabs.* (Yash) 1 tab thrice a day.
73. MIGRAINE	a. *Cephogran Tablets* (Charak) 1 tablet thrice a day.
	b. *Godanti Misram Tablet* 1 tablet twice daily.
	c. *Decil Tabs.* (J&J Dec.) 2 tablets twice a day.
	d. *Stresscom* (Dabur) *Caps.* 1 capsule twice a day.
74. MEMORY LOSS	a. *Brahmivati* (Dabur) 1 tab. twice daily.
	b. *B Vita Granules* 1 teaspoon with milk.
	c. *Tejras* (Sandu) 1 teaspoon twice a day.
	d. *Shankapushpi Syrup* (Baidyanath) 2 teaspoons twice a day.
	e. *Mentat Tabs.* (Himalaya) 1 tablet twice a day.
	f. *Vidhyaras Tablets* (Yash Ramadas) 1 tablet twice a day.

Complaint	Drugs
	g. *Memorin Caps.* (Phyto) 1 cap. twice a day.
	h. *Smrithi Granules* (Nagarjuna Keral) 1 teaspoonful mixed in milk twice a day.
	i. *Brahmivati Tabs.* (Unjah Pharmacy) 1 tab. twice a day.
	j. *Brento* (Zandu) *Tabs.* 2 tablets twice a day.
	k. *Vidyarthi Amritras* (Maharshi) 2 teaspoons twice a day.
75. MUMPS	a. *Septillin* (Himalaya) 2 tabs. twice a day.
	b. *Sallaki Tabs.* (GUFIC) 1 tablet twice a day.
	c. *Biogest Tabs.* (KAP) 1 tablet thrice a day.
76. MOUTH ULCERS (Stomatits)	a. *Kadiradi Vati* (Dabur) chew 1 to 6 tablets a day.
	b. *Triphala Churna* (Baidyanath) 3 tablespoons dissolve in a glassful of hot water and clean mouth twice a day.
77. NEURITIS	a. *Stress Nil Capsule* (Baidyanath) 1 capsule twice a day.
	b. *Rhuma Dap Tablets* 1 tablet twice a day.
	c. *Rumaflex Caps.* (Anuja) 1 capsule thrice a day.
	d. *Prasarini Tail* application (Baidyanath).
	e. *Actiflex Tabs.* (Anuja) 1 tablet thrice a day.
78. OBESITY	a. *Triphala Kada* (Sandu) 15 ml thrice a day with equal water.
	b. *Obenyl Tabs.* (Charak) 2 tablets twice a day.
	c. *Medohara Guggul* (Baidyanath) 2 pills twice a day.
	d. *Decrin Caps.* (Phyto) 1 capsule thrice a day.
	e. *Lipidsol Caps.* (Anuja) 1 capsule thrice a day.
	f. *Lipan Caps.* (BAN) 1 capsule twice a day.
79. PEPTIC ULCER	a. *Alsarex* (Charak) 2 tablets twice a day.
	b. *Sooktyn* (Alarsin) 1 tablet thrice a day.
	c. *Amlant Tab* (Maharshi) 1 tab thrice a day.
	d. *Soota Sekhar Tabs.* (Baidyanath) 1 tablet twice a day.
	e. *Kamadugdha Tabs.* (Shankar) 2 tablets thrice a day.
80. PILES	a. *Pilex* (Himalaya) *Tablets* and *Cream* 2 tablets thrice a day, cream for application.
	b. *Abhayarishta* (Dabur) 15 ml at bedtime with equal quantity of water.

Complaint	Drugs
	c. *Sunarin Caps.* (Phytopharma) 1 cap. thrice a day. d. *Piroids Tabs.* (Baidyanath) 1 tablet thrice a day. e. *Arshonyt* (Charak) *Tabs. & Ointment* 2 tabs. thrice a day. Apply ointment.
81. PROSTATE DISORDER	a. *Shilajitvadi Vati* (Baidyanath) 1 tablet thrice a day. b. *Chandra Prabha* (Zandu) 1 tablet twice a day. c. *Fortege* (Alarsin) *Tabs.* 2 tablets twice a day. d. *Bangshill* (Alarsin) *Tablets* 2 tabs. twice a day. e. *Shilajit Caps.* (Dabur) 1 cap twice a day.
82. PSORIASIS	a. *Oil 777* (Sidda) external application on the patches. b. *Epderm Caps.* (Capro-Banglore) 1 capsule twice a day. c. *Aarogyavardini* (Zandu) 1 tablet twice a day. d. *Pigmento* (Charak) 1 tablet twice a day. e. *Safi* (Hamdard) 2 teaspoons thrice a day.
83. PYORRHOEA	a. *Gumtone Powder* for regular application on gums. b. *Triphala Guggul* (Zandu) 2 pills twice a day. c. *Pyokill*-(Gurukul Kangdi) for ext. use on affected gums. d. *G-32 Tabs.* (Alarsin). Crush 2 tabs and apply on the gums.
84. PRICKLY HEAT	a. *Chandanadi Tail* (Baidyanath) for external application. b. *Saribadivati* (Baidyanath) 2 tabs. twice a day.
85. PLEURISY	a. *Laxmivilas ras* (Dabur) 1 tab. twice a day. b. Biogest (Kap) 2 tablets twice a day.
86. PUS IN THE EAR	a. Clean ear with lukewarm water and instill *Kshara Tail* (Baidyanath) 3 to 5 drops twice a day. b. *Saribadi Vati* (Badyanath) 1 tablet twice. c. *Septillin* (Himalaya) 2 tablets twice.
87. RHEUMATISM	a. *Simhanada Guggul* (Zandu) 2 pills twice a day. b. *Maha Rasnadi Kada* 15 ml twice daily with equal water. c. *Maha Narayana Tail* for external application. d. *Rumalaya Tablets* (Himalaya) 2 tablets twice a day. e. *R Pyrine* (Ban) Tablets 2 tabs twice a day. f. *Amavatari Ras* (Dabur) 2 pills twice a day. g. *Rheumat-90 Liquid* (Nagarjuna Kerala) 2 teaspoons thrice a day.

Complaint	Drugs
88. SINUSITIS	a. *Septillin Tablet* (Himalaya) 2 tablets twice a day. b. *Laxmi Vilas Tablet* (Dabur) 1 tablet twice a day.
89. STRESS	a. *Stress-nil Capsules* (Baidyanath) 1 capsule twice a day. b. *Stresscom* (Dabur) 1 capsule twice a day. c. *Bento Tabs.* (Zandu) 1 tablet twice a day. d. *Manasa Mitra* Vatakam (Arya Vaidyasala, Kerala) 1 tablet twice a day. e. *Bevibol Caps.* (Vasu, Gujrat) 1 capsule twice a day. f. *Alert Capsules* (Vasu) 1 capsule twice a day. g. *Mentat Tabs.* (Himalaya) 1 tablet twice a day. h. *Trasina Capsule* (Dey's) 1 capsule twice a day.
90. SCURVY	a. *Amlaki Rasayan* (Baidyanath) 1 teaspoon twice a day with milk. b. *Triphala Kada* (Sandu) 10 ml twice a day. c. *Amlaki Ghana Vati* (Chaitaya) 1 tab twice a day. d. *Charmon Drops* (BAN, Rajkot) 10 to 15 drops twice a day. e. *Chawanprasha* (Gurukul Kangdi) 1 tablespoon thrice a day.
91. SORE THROAT	a. *Khadiradi Vati* (Baidyanath) 1 tablet to be chewed as required. b. *Eladivati* (Baidyanath) 1 tablet thrice a day. c. *Septillin* (Himalaya) 1 tablet thrice a day. d. *Kachanara* (Zandu) 1 tablet thrice a day. e. *Kadiradi Vati* (Dabur) 1 tablet thrice chewable. f. *Talisapatradi Tablets* (Nagarjun Kerala) 2 tablets twice a day.
92. TONSILLITIS	a. *Septillin* (Himalaya) 2 tablets twice a day. b. *Kanchanara Guggul* (Zandu) 1 tab. thrice a day. c. *Decil Tabs.* (J&J Dechana Hyd) 2 tabs. twice a day. d. *Tonsikure Caps.* (Tansukh, Delhi) 1 capsule thrice a day. e. *Triphala Churna* (Baidyanath) 1 teaspoon with hot water at bed-time.
93. TOOTH-ACHE	a. *Lavanga Tail* (Dabur) for external application. b. *R. Compound* (Alarsin) 2 tablets twice a day.

Complaint	Drugs
94. UNDER-WEIGHT	a. *A.G. Forte* (Bajaj) 10 gms. twice a day with warm milk.
95. WHOOPING COUGH	b. *Tulsi Syrup* 10 ml twice a day.

2. REGIONAL NAMES OF SOME HERBS AND FRUITS

Sl. No.	SANSKRIT	HINDI	ENGLISH	LATIN	TELUGU	TAMIL
1.	ABHAYA	HARITAKI	CHEBULIC MYROBALAN	TERMINALIA CHEBULA	KARAKKAYYA	KADUKKA
2.	AJAMODA	AJMUDA	CELLARYSEEDS	CARUM AJMODA	AJAMODA	OMAM
3.	AKARAKARABHA	AKARKARA	PELLITORY ROOTS	ANACYCLUS PYRETHRUM	AKARAKARANA	AKKIRA-KARAMAI
4.	AMALAKI	AMLA	EMBELLIC MYROBALAN	PHYLLANTHUS EMBLICA	USIRIKAYA	NELLIKKAI
5.	AMRA	AM	MANGO	MANGIFERA INDICA	MAMIDI	MANGAI
6.	ANJIRA	ANJIR	FIG TREE	FICUS CARICA	SHIMI	ATTI/SHAMI
7.	ARISHTAKA	RITHA	SOAP NUT	SAPINDUS TRIFOLIATUS	KUNKIDI CHETTU	PUNNAN-KOTTAI
8.	ARJUNA	KAHUA	ARJUNA MYROBALAN	TERMINALIA ARJUNA	TELLAMADDI	BELMAI
9.	ASHOKA	ASHOK	ASHOKA TREE	SARACA INDICA	ASORAMU	ASOKAM
10.	ASHWAGANDHA	ASGANDH	WINTER CHERRY	WITHANIA SOMNIFERA	ASWAGANDHI	ASWAGANDHAI
11.	ATASI	ALSI	LINSEED	LINUM USITATISSIMUM	ATASI	ALISIDIRAI
12.	BABBULA	KIKAR	INDIAN GUM TREE	ACACIA ARABICA	NALLATHUMMA	KARUPEL
13.	BAKUCHI	BAKUCHI	BABCHI	PSORALIA CORYLIFOLIA	BAMANCHI	KARPOKARISI
14.	BHALLATAKA	BHILAWA	MARKINGNUT	SEMICARPUS ANACARDIUM	BHALLATHAKA	SENGOTTAI
15.	BHRINGARAJA	BHANGRA	MARKINGNUT	ECLIPTA ALBA	GALAGARA	KAIKESI
16.	BILWA	BAEL	BAEL	AEGLE MARMELOS	BILWAM	VILWAM
17.	BIMBI	TRIKOL		COCCINIA INDICA	DONDAKAYA	KOVAKKAI
18.	BRAHMI	BRAHMI	INDIAN PENNYWORT	BACOPA MONNIERI	SAMBRANICHETTU	NEERBRAHMI
19.	CHANDANA	CHANDAN	SANDALWOOD	SANTALUM ALBUM	CHANDANAM	SANDANAM
20.	CHITRAKA	CHITRAK	LEADWORT	PLUMBAGO ZEYLANICA	CHITTIRAM	TELLACHITRA

Sl. No.	SANSKRIT	HINDI	ENGLISH	LATIN	TELUGU	TAMIL
21.	CHOPCHINI	CHOBCHINI	CHINAROOT	SMILAX CHINA	PHIRANGI CHEKKA	PARANGI-CHEKKAI
22.	DADIMA	ANAR	POMEGRANATE	PUNICA GRANATUM	DANNIMMA	MATHAL NARANGAI
23.	DEVADARU	DEVDAR	DEODAR	CEDRUS DEODARA	DEVADARU	DEVADARU
24.	DHANYAKA	DHANIYA	CORIANDER	CORIANDRUM SATIVUM	DHANIYALU	KOTHAMALLI
25.	DRAKSHA	DRAKSH	GRAPES	VITIS VINIFERA	DRAKSHAPANDU	DRATCHAI
26.	ELA	ELAICHI	CARDAMOM	ELETTARIA CARDAMOMUM	ELAKKAI	ELAKKAI
27.	KUMARI	GHRITKUMARI	ALOE	ALOW VERA	KALABANDHA	CHIRULI
28.	ERANDA KARKATI	PAPAYA	PAPAYA TREE	CARICA PAPAYA	PAPAYA	PAPAYA
29.	ERANDMOOL	ARAND	CASTOR (OIL TREE)	RICINUS COMMUNIS	AMADAM CHETTU	AVANAKKU
30.	GAJAPIPPALI	GAJPIPAL	ELEPHANT PIPER	SCINDAPSUS OFFICIALIS	GAJAPIPPALLU	
31.	GOJIHWA	GHOZA-BAN/ SANKHAHUL		ONOSMA BRACTEATUM		
32.	GARJARA	GAJAR	CARROT	DAUCAS CAROTA	-	-
33.	GOKSHURA	GOKHRU BARA	CALTROPS	TRIBULUS TERRESTRIS	PALLERU MULLU	NYERINGILMUL
34.	GUGGULU	GUGAL	INDIAN BEDELLIUM	COMMIPHORA MUKUL	GUGGILAM	GUKKULU
35.	GUDUCHI	GILOY		TINOSPORA CORDIFOLIA	THIPPATHEEGA	SEENTHILRODI
36.	HARIDRA	HALDI	TURMERIC	CURCUMA LONGA	PASUPU	MANJAL
37.	HINGU	HING	ASAFOETIDA	FERULA FOETIDA	INGUVA	KAYAM
38.	HINGUPATRI	DIKAMALI	WHITE EMETIC NUT	PEUCADANUM GRANDE		
39.	IKSHU	UKH	SUGARCANE	SACCHARUM OFFICINARUM	CHERUKU	KARUMBU
40.	JAMBU	JAMUN	BLACK PLUM	EUGENIA JAMBOLANA	NERUDU	NAVAL
41.	JAMBIRA	JAMIRI NIMBU	LEMON	CITRUS MEDICA	NIMMA	ELIMICHAM
42.	JATAMAMSI	BALCHAD	MUSKROOT	NORDOSTACHYS JATAMAMSI	JATAMAMSI	JADAMANSI
43.	JATIPHALA	JAIPHAL	NUTMEG	MYRSTICA FRAGRANS	JAJIKAYA	JATHIKKAI

Sl. No.	SANSKRIT	HINDI	ENGLISH	LATIN	TELUGU	TAMIL
44.	JATIPATRI	JAVITRI	MACE	MYRSTICA FRAGRANS	JAJIKAYA	JATHIKKAI
45.	JIRAKA	JEERA	CUMIN SEED	CUMINUM CYMINUM	JEELAKARRA	JEERAKAM
46.	JYOTISHMATI	MALKANGNI	STAFF TREE	CELASTRUS PANNICULATUS		VALULAVAI
47.	KABABCHINI	KABABCHINI	CUBEB	PIPER CUBEBA	THOKAMIRIYAM	VALMILAGU
48.	KADALI	KELA	BANANA	MUSA SAPIENTUM	ARATI	VAZHAI
49.	KAKAMACHI	MAKA	BLACK NIGHTSHADE	SOLANUM NIGER	KACHIPANDU	MANTHA KKALI
50.	KANCHANAR	KACHNAR	THE CREAT	BAUHINIA VARIEGATA	DEVAKANCHANAM	MANDARAI
51.	KAPIKACHU	KIWANCH	COWHAGE PLANT	MUCUNA PRURIENS	PILLIYADUGU	PUNNAIKKALI
52.	KAPITHA	KAITH	WOOD APPLE	FERIONIA ELEPHANTUM	KAPITHA	
53.	KARPURA	KAPOOR	CAMPHOR	CINNAMOMUM CAMPHORA	KARPOORAM	KARPOORAM
54.	KARAVIRA	KANER	INDIAN OLEANDER	NERIUM INDICUM	GANNERU	ARALI
55.	KATUKI	KUTKI	HELL BORE	PICRORHIZA KURROA	KATUKAROHINI	KADUGA ROHINI
56.	KETAKI	KEWRA	KEORA / SCREW PINE	PANDANUS ODORITISSIMUS	MOGALI	JAVANANA
57.	KHARJURA	KHAJUR	DATE PALM	PHOENIX DACTYLIFERA	KHARJURAKKAI	
58.	KHADIRA	KHADIR SWET	CATECHU CUTCH-TREE	ACACIA SENEGAL	SANDRA	KARANGALLI
59.	KIRATHATIKTA	CHIRAITA	CHIRETTA	SWERTIA CHIRATA	NILAVEMU	NILAVEMBU
60.	KRISHNA JIRAKA	SYAHA JIRA	CARAWAY SEEDS/BLACK CARAWAY	CARUM CARVI	SEEMAJEELAKARRA	SEEMAI-JEERAGAM
61.	KUBERAKSHI	LATAKARANJA	BONDU / FEVER NUT	CAESALPINIA CRISTA	GACHAKAI	KAJUKKAI
62.	KUMKUMA	KESHAR	SAFFRON	CROCUS SATIVUS	KUNKUMAPUVVU	KUNGU-MAPPOO
63.	KUSHTA	KUTH	COSTUS	SAUSSUREA LAPPA	KUSTHAM	KOTTAM
64.	KUTAJA	KURCHI/ KUDA	CONESSI BARK	HOLARRHENA ANTI DYSENTERICA	KODAGA	VEPPALLAI
65.	LAJJALU	LAJWANTI	SENSITIVE PLANT/ TOUCH ME NOT	MIMOSA PUDICA	ATTAPATHI	THOTTALVADI

Sl. No.	SANSKRIT	HINDI	ENGLISH	LATIN	TELUGU	TAMIL
66.	LAKSHA	L`AKSA	LAC	COCCULUS LACK	LAKKA	
67.	LASUNA	LEHSUN	GARLIC	ALLIUM SATIVUM	VELLULLI	POONDU
68.	LAVANGA	LONG	CLOVE	EUGENIA CARYOPHYLLATA	LAVANGAM	LAVANGAM
69.	LODHRA	LODHRA	LODHRA	SYMPLOCOS RACEMOSA	LODHUGA	VELLILEDI
70.	LOHBAN	LOBAN	BENZOIN	STYRAX BENZOIN	SAMBRANI	SAMBRANI
71.	MAHANIMBA	BAKAYAN	BEAD TREE	MELIA AZARIDACH	TIRUKAVEPPA	MALAIVEMBU
72.	MANJISHTA	MAJEETH	MADDER ROOT	RUBIA CORDIFOLIA	TAMRAVALLI	MANJITTI
73.	MARICHA	KALIMIRCH	BLACK PEPR	PIPER NIGRUM	MIRIYALU	MELAGU
74.	MARKANDI	SONAMUKHI	SENNA	CASSIA AUGUSTIFOLIA		
75.	MARICHA (RAKTA)	LALMIRCH	RED CHILLY	CAPSICUM FRUITESCENS	MIRAPAKAYA	MOLAGA
76.	MADAYANTIKA	MEHNDI	HENNA	LAWSONIA INERMIS	GORANTA	MARUDHANI
77.	METHIKA	METHI	FENUGREEK	TRIGONELLA FOENUM GRAECUM	MENTHULU	VENDHAYAM
78.	MOOLAKA	MULI	RADISH	RAPHANUS SATIVUS		
79.	MUSALI	MUSLI		ASPARAGUS ADSCENDENS	NELATIDI CHETTU/GADDA	NEELAPANAI
80.	MUSTA	MOTHA	NUTGRASS	CYPRUS ROTUNDUS	THUNGAMUSTA	MUNTHANGAI/ KORAKKI-ZHANGU
81.	MUNDI	MUNDI	NUTGRASS	SPHAERANTHUS INDICUS	VODDATHARUPU	KOAI
82.	NADIHINGU	DIKAMALI	GUMMY GARDENIA	GARDENIA GUMMIFERA		
83.	NARIKELA	NARIYAL	COCONUT	COCUS NUCIFERA	KOBBARI	THENGAI
84.	NIMBUKA	KAGJI NIMBU	LEMON	CITRUS ACIDA	NIMMA	
85.	NIRGUNDI	SAMBHALU	FINE LEAVED CHASTE	VITEX NIGUNDO	TELLAVAVILI	NOCHI
86.	VATA	BAT	BANYAN TREE	FICUS BENGALENSIS	MARRI	AALAMARAM
87.	PADMA	KAMAL	LOTUS	NELUMBIUM SPECIOSUM	KALUVA	THAMARAI
88.	PADMAKA	PADMA KAST	HIMALAYAN CHERRY	PRUNUS CARASOIDES		
89.	PALANDU	PYAZ	ONION	ALLIUM CEPA	ULLIPAYA	VENGAYAM

Sl. No.	SANSKRIT	HINDI	ENGLISH	LATIN	TELUGU	TAMIL
90.	PARASEEKA YAVANI	KHURASANI AJWAIN	HENBANE	HYOSCYAMUS NIGER		
91.	PATOLA	PARVAL	WILD SNAKE GOURD	TRICHOSANTHES DIOICA	POTLAKAYA	PODALANGAI
92.	PIPPALI	PIPLA	LONG PEPPER	PIPER LONGUM	PIPPALLU	THIPPALAI
93.	PIPPALIMULA	PIPLAMOOLA		ROOTS OF PIPER LONGUM		
94.	POOGI	SUPARI	BETEL NUT	ARECA CATECHU	VAKKA	PAKKU
95.	PUNARNAVA (RAKTA)	PUNAR NAVA	SPREADING HOGWEED	BOERRHAVIA DIFFUSA	ATTAMAMIDI	MURUKKATTA/ THALUDAMAI
96.	RAKTHA NIRYASA	KHOON KHARABA	INDIAN KINO	CALAMUS DRACO		
97.	RASNA	RASNA		VANDA ROXBURGHII		
98.	RAKTHACHANDAN	LALCHANDAN	RED SANDAL	PTEROCARPUS SANTALINUS	RAKTACHANDANAM	RATHA-CHANDANAM
99.	RUDRAKSHA	RUDRAKSHA		ELAEOCARPUS GANITRUS	RUDRAKSHA	RUDRATCHAI
100.	SAPTAPARNI	CHATIMLEGHI	DITA	ALSTONIA SCHOLARIS	EDAKULARITA	EZHILAMPALAI
101.	SARPAGANDHA	CHOTA CHAND		RAUWOLFIA SERPENTINA	PATALAGANI	CHIVANA-MELPODI
102.	SHANKHPUSHPI	SANKAHURI		CONVOLVULUS PLEURICAULIS		
103.	SHARAPUNKHA	SARPHOUNKA	PURPLE TEPHROSIA	TEPHROSIA PURPURA	VEMPALLI	KOLINGI
104.	SHATAMULI	SHATAVRI	ASPARAGUS	ASPARAGUS RACEMOSUS	PILLI THUGA KIZHANGU	THANEER VITTAN
105.	SHATAPUSHPA	SAUNFBARI	FENNEL/DILL	FOENICULUM VULGARIS	SHATAKUPPI VITTALU	SHATAKUPPI-VERU
106.	SHOBHANJANA	SONJNA	DRUMSTICK TREE	MORINGA OLEIFERA	MUNAKKAI	MURUN-GAKKAI
107.	SHIRISHA	SIRIS		ALBIZZIA LEBBECK	DIRASANA	VEGAI
108.	SURANJANA	SURANJAN TALICH	COLCHICUM	COLCHICUM LUTEUM		

3. METHODS OF HERBAL PREPARATION

1. **INFUSION:** Similar to tea preparation. This may be hot/cold.

a) **Hot:** One tablespoon of herb (5gm approximately) is added to a glass full of boiling water, covered with a lid and allowed to seep into the water for 10-15 minutes. This mixture is later filtered with a clean muslin cloth and used.
   Note:
   1. One part of dried herb can be replaced by 3 parts of the fresh herb.
   2. Infusion should be drunk hot and freshly prepared.
   3. The dry herb should be powdered to release the volatile oils from the cells before use.
   4. Aluminium vessels are avoided for best results.

b) **Cold:** The preparation is similar to the above, except that cold water is used instead of hot water and the infusion is left to seep for 6-12 hours in a well sealed earthen pot after which it is filtered and used.
   Note: This process is adopted where the herbs are more sensitive to heat and contain highly volatile oils.

2. **DECOCTION:** One tablespoon of dried herb (or 3 tablespoons of crushed herb) is added to a glass full of water in a vessel and heated till boiling for about 10-15 minutes (until the water is reduced to half the original quantity). It is then filtered with a clean muslin cloth and used when still hot.
   Note: This procedure is especially adopted when the herb used is hard or woody, e.g. rhizomes, barks, nuts etc.

3. **POWDER:** Dried raw drugs are made into microfine powder and stored dry. The shelf life for such powders is 6 months.

4. **PASTE:** Raw drugs are ground with water or specified liquid to paste-like consistency. This must be used fresh everyday.

5. **JUICE:** Raw drugs crushed with a little water are squeezed through a fresh cloth to obtain the juice. Even this is prepared and used afresh everyday.

6. **OIL/GHEE:** Method of preparation of oil and *ghee* is the same except for obviously, the base material (cow's *ghee* is generally implied in the *ghee* preparations). 1 kg of the *ghee*/oil.
   4 kg of raw drug decoction and 250 grams of the paste of raw drugs are mixed in a vessel and boiled until all the water content is evaporated.

INDICATIONS OF STOPPAGE OF PROCEDURE

1. Appearance of bubbles/foam on the surface of oil. Disappearance of bubbles/foam on the surface of ghee.
2. a) If for external use, the paste in the preparation should have turned dry.
   b) If for internal use, the paste added in the vessel should be muddy in nature.
   c) If for the use of nasal drops, the paste added should be thready in nature.
7. **Herbal Ointment:** The commonly used base is petroleum jelly/bees wax or medicated oil.
   1. The drugs are first made into an infusion or decoction of 500 ml, filtered and kept aside.
   2. 90 ml of the base (oil, petroleum jelly etc.) is poured into a pan and heated on low fire along with the prepared decoction/infusion until the watery components evaporate completely and the extract has blended completely with the base. Stir until semisolid consistency is attained. Allow to cool and store.

Note:
1. Care should be taken not to overheat the mixture.
2. Indication of complete evaporation of water is the stoppage of bubble appearance.

4. GLOSSARY OF MEDICAL TERMS USED

1. **Anthelmintics:** These are medicines/drugs which kill, expel or prevent the return of worms.
2. **Antiseptics:** These are agents/drugs which prevent, retard or arrest putrifaction.
3. **Antipyretics:** These are agents/drugs which reduce temperature.
4. **Antispasmodics:** These are the class of drugs which prevent or allay the irregular muscular contractions called spasms or cramps.
5. **Aphrodisiacs:** These are the group of drugs which increase sexual desire and stimulate the functions of the genital organs.
6. **Astringents:** These are the agents/drugs which contract muscular tissue, promote the coagulation of fluids and check secretions.
7. **Aromatics:** These are the drugs/agents which possess an agreeable taste and colour.
8. **Carminatives:** These are drugs/agents which are capable of expelling gas from the alimentary canal and remove pain.

9. **Demulcents/Emmolients:** Agents which soften the part to which they are applied and diminish irritation. When used externally to protect the mucous membranes of the alimentary canal from the action of irritants, they are termed demulcents.
10. **Disinfectants:** These are agents, which render infectious matter inert.
11. **Diuretics:** These are drugs which cause an increased secretion and discharge of urine.
12. **Digestives:** Drugs or agents which assist digestion.
13. **Emmollients:** See Demulcents.
14. **Emmenogogues:** These are agents which stimulate the action of the uterus and directly assist in correcting disordered menstruation.
15. **Expectorants:** These are the drugs/agents which cause the expulsion of bronchial secretions.
16. **Hypotensives:** The drugs which cause fall of blood pressure are called hypotensives.
17. **Narcotics:** The agents/drugs which allay pain and induce sleep.
18. **Rubefacients:** Agents/drugs which when applied to the skin irritate and redden it.
19. **Sedatives:** Agents which depress the nervous system and produce sleep.
20. **Stimulants:** Agents which rapidly excite the nervous system to increase activity.
21. **Stomachics:** Agents which increase the vascularity of the stomach, promote digestion and increase appetite.
22. **Vermifuges:** See anthelmentics.
23. **Vitalizers:** Agents which promote vitality.

5. THERAPEUTIC DIETS

The following are some important diets recommended by the National Institute of Nutrition, Hyderabad.

I. BLAND DIET

A bland diet is a diet which is non-irritating chemically and mechanically and which inhibits gastric secretion, can be used for gastric and duodenal ulcer patients with slight modifications and a reduction in fibre and fat content. It can also be used for diarrhoea and ulcerative colitis.

Principle: The following foods should be **avoided** while formulating the diet.

1. Bran and coarse cereals
2. Skin and seeds of fruits
3. Raw vegetables
4. Vegetables like cabbage, bean, ladies finger and bittergourd etc.
5. Spices and condiments
6. Fried foods
7. Strong beverages
8. Pickles, chutneys etc.
9. Chocolates, puddings and similar preparations
10. Meat extracts and soups.

II. SAMPLE DIET (NON-PRESCRIBED)

Food stuff	Vegetarian (g)
Rice	100 gm
White Bread	40 gm
Pulses	40 gm
Potatoes	75 gm
Vegetables	100 gm
Milk	1000 ml
Yoghurt	300 ml

Contd....

Skimmed Milk Powder	15 gm
Orange Juice	150 ml
Banana	50 gm
Sugar	25 gm
Butter	7 gm
Ghee or oil	25 ml*

Note: Non-vegetarians can take a half boiled egg instead of skimmed milk powder.

*This amount can be used for cooking purposes. This diet provides:

Calories   -   2000
Proteins   -   75g
Fats   -   90g
Carbohydrates - 220g

III. DIABETIC DIET (PRESCRIBED DIET)

This diet is very close to the normal diet so as to meet the nutritional needs and the treatments of the individual patient. This diet is slightly low in carbohydrates but adequate in other food principles.

Principle:
The following foods should be avoided in all diabetic diets:
1. Roots and tubers
2. Sweets, puddings and chocolates
3. Fried foods
4. Dried fruits and nuts
5. Sugar
6. Fruits like banana, sapota, custard apple etc.

Food stuff	Vegetarian (gm)	Non-vegetarian (gm)
Cereals	200	250
Pulses	60	20
Green-leafy vegetables	200	200
Other vegetables	200	200
Fruits	200	200
Milk (Dairy)	400	200
Oil	20	20
Fish/Chicken without skin	-	100

This diet provides:

Calories	1600
Proteins	65 gm
Fat	40 gm
Carbohydrates	245 gm

Distribution:

	Cooking measures Vegetarian	Non-vegetarian
Bed Tea		
Coffee or tea	1 Cup	1 Cup
Breakfast		
Toast with a little butter	1 No.	1 No.
Coffee or tea	1 Cup	1 Cup
Lunch		
Rice	2 Katories	2 Katories
Sambar	1 Katori	1 Katori
Green-leafy vegetables	1 Katori	1 Katori
Curd	1/2 Katori	1/2 Katori
Tomato or citrus fruits	1 No.	1 No.
Pickle	a piece	a piece
Tiffin		
Tea or coffee	1 Cup	1 Cup
Upma	3/4 Katori	1 Katori
Dinner		
Phulka (Chapati)	3 No.	4 Nos.
Dal	1 Katori	-
Curd	1/2 Katori	-
Fish/Chicken	-	2 pieces
Other vegetables with gravy	1 Katori	1 Katori
Roasted papad	1 No.	1 No.
Tomato or cucumber	1 No.	1 No.
Before going to bed		
Milk	1 Cup	1 Cup

Note: 5 teaspoons of oil can be used in cooking.

IV. LOW-CALORIE DIET

The diet provides less calories than the total energy requirements for the day; thus it provides for depletion of body fats. It is used in cases of obesity, cardiac disturbances and hypertension in overweight individuals.

Principle:

The following foods should be avoided while formulating the diet:
1. Sweets, chocolates, jaggery, jam, honey, preservatives, puddings, cakes etc.
2. Roots and tubers
3. Fried foods
4. Dried fruits and nuts
5. Alcoholic drinks and soft drinks unless they contain artificial sweetening agents instead of sugar
6. Cream and free fats
7. Fruits like banana, custard-apple, sapota, dates etc.

Sample Diet:

Food stuff	Vegetarian (gm)	Non-vegetarian (gm)
Wheat flour	60	60
Rice	30	60
Other vegetables	200	200
Green-leafy vegetables	200	200
Pulses	70	50
Citrus fruits or tomato	200	200
Milk (cow's)	600 ml	250 ml
Skimmed milk powder	20	–
Oil or ghee	7	12
Lean meat or fish	–	50
Egg	–	One

This diet provides:

Calories	1200
Proteins	60 gm
Fat	30 gm
Carbohydrates	170 gm

V. HIGH-CALORIE DIET

This is a normal diet supplemented with high calorie foods so that the bulk of the diet is not much increased. It can be used for fevers, convalescence after prolonged illness, leanness and hyperthyroidism.

Principle:

The following foods should be avoided if the patient is convalescing or having fever:
1. Fried foods.
2. Dry fruits and nuts.

Sample Diet:

Food stuff	Weight of raw ingredients	
	Vegetarian (gm)	Non-vegetarian (gm)
Cereals	250	300
Pulses	100	50
Roots and tubers	50	75
Other vegetables	50	50
Green leafy vegetables	100	100
Bread	60	60
Butter	10	20
Milk	750 ml	300 ml
Curd	100	-
Sugar	50	50
Ghee/oil	30	30
Banana	150	250
Egg	-	One
Meat or fish	-	100

This diet provides:

Calories	2700
Proteins	80 gm
Fats	70 gm

VI. LOW FAT DIET

This is a normal diet modified to reduce the fat content to approximately 30g per day. It may be used in treating diseases with intolerance to fat such as gall bladder, liver and pancreatic diseases or in conditions of steatorrhoea.

Principle:

The following foods should be avoided in such diets:

1. High fat foods like nuts, cheese etc.
2. Fried foods
3. Free fat and cream etc.

Sample Diet:

Food stuff	Vegetarian (gm)	Non-vegetarian (gm)
Cereals	200	250
Pulses	100	75
Cow's milk	-	100 ml
Skimmed milk powder	50	-
Curd (cow's milk)	200	-
Green leafy vegetables	100	100
Other vegetables	100	100
Potatoes	50	50
Sugar	50	50
Banana	75	75
Orange	100	100
Ghee or oil to cook	17	15
Chicken or fish	-	100
Eggs	-	One

This diet provides:

Calories	2100
Proteins	75 gm
Fats	30 gm
Carbohydrates	385 gm

VII. LOW CHOLESTEROL AND REDUCED SATURATED FAT DIET

This is a normal diet formulated with increased polyunsaturated fats. It is adequate in all nutrients. It can help to lower plasma cholesterol. Amount of calories and proteins can be changed with individual needs.

Principle:

The following foods should be avoided while formulating the diet.

1. Butter, hydrogenated fat and lard
2. Coconut and coconut oil
3. Foods cooked with these fats
4. Fatty meat, visible fat on meat, sausages etc.
5. Whole milk and cream
6. Chocolate and ice-cream
7. Cheese
8. Organ meats like liver, kidney and brain etc.
9. Shrimp
10. Eggs, only two per week.

Sample Diet:

Food stuff	Quantity (gm)
Cereals	300
Pulses	50
Green-leafy vegetables	50
Other vegetables	100
Roots and tubers	100
Fruits	100
Skimmed milk	400
Sugar	30
Oil	30

This diet provides:

Calories	2400
Proteins	70 gm
Fats	55 gm
Carbohydrates	400 gm

VIII. LOW SODIUM DIET FOR HYPERTENSION

This is a normal diet but with a low sodium content. The food preparations for this diet are cooked without extra salt and high sodium foods are avoided. This is designed for use in conditions where there is sodium reaction like oedema, nephritis, cardiac diseases, toxaemia of pregnancy and hypertension.

Principle:

The following foods should be avoided:

1. Salt in cooking or on table.
2. Sea fish, salted meat and salted dry fish, liver etc.
3. Salted butter and cheese.
4. All foods to which salt or baking soda has been added in cooking.
5. Pickles and chutneys.

Food stuff	Vegetarian (gm)	Non-vegetarian (gm)
Rice	250	300
Dal	100	75
Fruits	200	200
Vegetables	200	200
Potatoes	100	125
Milk (cow's)	600 ml	200 ml
Oil	30	30
Sugar	30	50
Meat or fish		50
Eggs		one

This diet provides:

Calories	2200
Proteins	70 gm
Sodium (as sodium)	0.5 gm

IX. LOW OXALIC ACID DIET

This is a normal diet with a low oxalic acid content. High oxalic acid foods are avoided. This is designed for use by the patients suffering from oxalate calculi.

Principle:

Foods rich in oxalic acid should be avoided.

Sample Diet:

Food stuff	Vegetarian (gm)	Non-vegetarian (gm)
Rice	200	200
Wheat flour	200	200
Red gram dal	50	35
Black gram dal	20	20
Cabbage	100	100
Potato	75	75
Mango	75	75
Milk	200 ml	100 ml
Oil	35	40
Sugar	30	30
Mutton or Rohu fish	-	30
Egg	-	30

This diet provides:

Calories	2400
Proteins	65 gm
Fats	50 gm
Carbohydrates	425 gm

X. LIQUID DIET

This diet is designed to give oral nourishment in the liquid form. It can be used for the patients who cannot tolerate or consume solid or semi-solid foods. Since this diet does not provide enough nutrients, it should not be continued for more than necessary time.

Sample Diet:

Food Stuff	Quantity
Milk	1000 ml
Fruit juice	1000 ml
Eggs	Two
Sugar	50 gm

This diet provides:

Calories	1400
Proteins	52g
Calcium	1760 mg
Iron	11.1 mg
Retinol	1100 micro mg
Thiamin	1.4 mg
Riboflavin	1.8 mg

XI. DIET FOR PREGNANT WOMAN

This diet provides slightly higher amounts of proteins, calories, minerals and vitamins than required for a normal woman. It can be given to a pregnant woman in the second and third trimesters of pregnancy when there is extra demand for these nutrients because of the developing foetus.

Principle: All the food stuffs available to the family can be taken by a pregnant woman. There is no specific restriction on any food stuff.

Sample Diet:

Food stuff	Sedentary work vegetarian (gm)	Moderate work vegetarian (gm)
Cereals	445	475
Pulses	55	60
Green-leafy vegetables	100	100
Other vegetables	40	40
Roots and tubers	50	50
Milk	200 ml	250 ml
Fats and oils	20	20
Sugar and jaggery	30	30

This diet provides:

Calories	2200	2500
Proteins	70 gm	75 gm
Fats	40 gm	50 gm

Non-vegetarians can substitute the pulses with 2 eggs or 50gm of meat or fish, plus 10gm of fat.

XII. DIET FOR NURSING MOTHER

This diet provides slightly more of all nutrients than what are required by a normal woman. It can be used by a nursing mother, throughout her lactation period. All the food stuffs available can be consumed by a lactating mother. There is no specific taboo on any food stuff.

Sample Diet

Food stuff	Sedentary work vegetarian (gm)	Moderate work vegetarian (gm)
Cereals	470	500
Pulses	70	75
Green leafy vegetables	100	100
Other Vegetables	40	40
Roots and Tubers	50	50
Milk	200 ml	250 ml
Fats and Oils	30	35
Sugar and Jaggery	30	30

This diet provides:

Calories	2450	2750
Proteins	75 gm	80 gm
Fats	50 gm	60 gm

Non-vegetarians can substitute pulses with 2 eggs or 50 gm of meat or fish, plus 10gm of fats.

FOODS RICH IN OXALIC ACID

Horse gram	Rhubarb (Stalk)
Khesari dal	Almonds
Amaranth, tender	Cashew nuts
Curry leaves	Garden cress seeds
Drumstick leaves	*Amla*
Gogu (Pitwa or ambadi)	*Phalsa*
Mustard leaves, tender	Wood apple

Contd....

Neem leaves, tender	Bhangari
Paruppu kerai (Kulfa)	*Chookri-ka-atla*
Spinach	*Chookri-ka-patla*
Tamarind leaves, tender	Ripe chillies
Drumstick leaves	Cocoa
Lotus stem, dry	Tea
Plantain flower	
Plantain green	

BIBLIOGRAPHY

1. A to Z Medical Hand Book — BLHZ Editions (1991).
2. First Aid Manual — St. John Ambulance, Red Cross Society, London.
3. Therapeutic Diets — National Institute of Nutrition, Hyderabad.
4. The Healing Arts — T.E.D. Kaptchuk and Michael Crouchor, BBC Publication, 1986, London
5. The Himalaya Drug Co., Bangalore, Periodical Publications.
6. The Readers Digest.
7. Therapeutic Guide to Ayurveda — Baidyanath Publication.
8. Indian Materia Medica volume — Nadkarni
9. Dravya guna vignan — P.V.Sharma, Chowkhamba Orientalia, Varanasi.
10. Indian Medicinal Plants — Nadkarni.
11. The Complete Illustrated Holistic Herbal — Elements Books Ltd., Great Britain 1996.

Green Remedies

—*Dr. S. Suresh Babu*
Dr. M. Madhavi

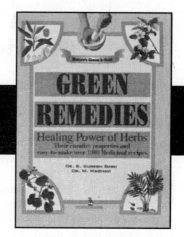

"**G**reen is Gold" is the global buzz-word, nowadays. Rediscover the remarkable curative powers of vital herbs. This indispensable lead book chronicles about 80 green resources and over 600 simplified herbal recipes that are proven cures for a large number of frequently encountered ailments and common health problems. Indeed, green remedies are the most sought-after solutions for safe health management, preferred by all advanced Western nations.

This superb book captures the spirit of Ayurveda and renders a true gist of its grand treatise. It lucidly enunciates the quintessence of herbal medicinal knowledge and applied treatments, as embodied and propounded by the masters of yore, like sages Charaka and Sushruta.

The book addresses the immediate health problems of the common man. The authors' efforts are directed solely to awaken the minds of masses, calling for sensible approach to the simple herbal medicines that are immensely effective, safe and reasonable for all practical purposes. Needless to say, all medicinal recipes discussed are wholly based on sound ayurvedic medical texts.

Big Size • Pages: 244
Price: Rs. 175/- • Postage: Rs. 20/-

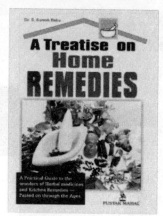

A Treatise on
Home Remedies

—Dr. S. Suresh Babu, M.D. (Ayur)

A practical guide to the wonders of herbal medicines and kitchen remedies—passed on through the Ages.

Modern medical science may be effective in treating a variety of diseases, but often fails when it comes to chronic problems like gastric-disorders, common cold, respiratory ailments and many others. Here the positive role of traditional, ayurvedic and herbal and home medicines has been proven beyond doubt.

This volume brings you an overview of specific problems—backed by not only ayurvedic remedies but also home remedies, along with dietary restrictions and dos & don'ts. From flatulence, constipation, cirrhosis of liver to hepatitis, jaundice and common cold—it covers a broad range. For instance, how a peptic ulcer is formed, and how cold milk is useful in providing relief. Or what are the problems accompanying dysentery and how the 'Bel' fruit is effective in its treatment.

The unique feature of the book is the treatment through home remedies—items which we've always had at hand in our kitchen like *haldi*, *methi*, coconut, cumin (*jeera*), clove, castor etc. What's more—additional treatments in the form of medicated massages, Hydrotherapy through fomentation methods and home beauty aids also bring you useful tips for a healthy and happy life.

Big Size • Pages: 220 • Price: Rs. 150/- • Postage: Rs. 25/-

Nature Cure at Home
Towards Better Health

—Dr. Rajeshwari

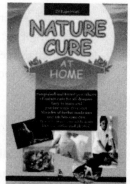

Public awareness of health is increasing day by day. Health guides and articles are in great demand as people are eager to learn about diseases, their prevention and ways of staying fit, without seeking any medical help. This quest, in part, is due to the realisation that diseases are more easily prevented than cured. This is an encouraging trend.

The author, Dr. Rajeshwari has an illustrious record of practising in several fields of alternative medicines like Naturopathy, Acupressure, Acupuncture, Yoga, Homeopathy and Magnetotherapy.

The book is written for those readers who would like to take care of their own health, using simple remedies, exercises and dietary measures, without exposing themselves to the dangerous side - effects and reactions of potent drugs.

It explains: ❖ Simplified yet effective procedures of nature cure ❖ Herbal remedies for effective treatment of diseases ❖ Curative powers of water.

Demy Size • Pages: 232 • Price: Rs. 80/- • Postage: Rs. 25/-

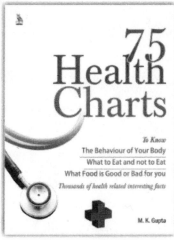

Price: Rs. 120/-
Big Size • Pages: 264

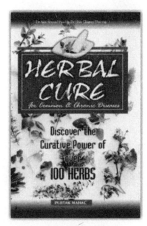

Price: Rs. 88/-
Demy Size • Pages: 152

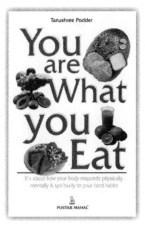

Price: Rs. 96/-
Demy Size • Pages: 184

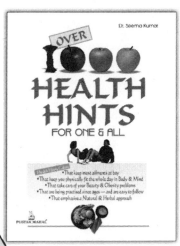

Price: Rs. 96/-
Big Size • Pages: 168

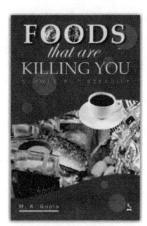

Price: Rs. 96/-
Demy Size • Pages: 160

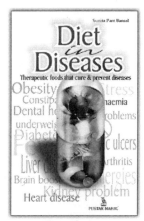

Price: Rs. 69/-
Demy Size • Pages: 104